The Good Teeth Guide

JOHN FORREST

Second Edition

GRANADA
London Toronto Sydney New York

Granada Publishing Limited
8 Grafton Street, London W1X 3LA

Published by Granada Publishing 1981
Second edition 1985

British Library Cataloguing in Publication Data

Forrest, John
   The good teeth guide. 2nd ed.
   1. Teeth – Care and hygiene
   I. Title
   617.6'01   RK61

ISBN 0 246 12695 7 ✓ß

Printed in Great Britain by
Richard Clay (The Chaucer Press) Ltd,
Bungay, Suffolk

Contents

Preface

This book sets out to explain modern dentistry. It also provides the information you need about obtaining dental *attention* (I prefer not to use the term 'treatment'). Very few books have been written for the general public about dental problems and their resolution, since dentists are not in general good communicators and may not like to lose the medical 'mystique' which they think sets them apart from the masses. But explaining often removes a great deal of worry and so I have discussed all the major problems that occur in adults and children, not only in respect of the teeth, but of other areas of the mouth and jaws which must be regarded as an integral unit.

Throughout the book I lay emphasis on the importance of preventing oral disease and describe correct home care by the subject or by his or her parents, a regime which must always be supported by regular visits to the dentist.

In view of my advocacy of preventive dentistry, it may be surprising that so large a proportion of the book is devoted to the problems and care of artificial dentures. As, however, dentures are the most frequent cause of dissension between dentist and patient, and as there are about one hundred million denture wearers in the English-speaking countries, it would be unfair to ignore an area of dentistry which regrettably still absorbs a good deal of time and money. With greater knowledge and care the proportion of denture wearers will be considerably reduced in succeeding generations.

This is not intended to be a 'do it yourself' dentistry book. The reader is directed to expert advice wherever and whenever possible. However, I do give advice on what to do in an emergency so that there will be no deterioration before the expert can be seen.

I have gone to great lengths not to take sides. No attack is made either on the patient or on the dental profession. I have, on the contrary, taken pains to illustrate the difficult job that dentists do and, on the whole, do very well indeed.

There has always seemed to me to be a love-hate relationship between patient and dentist. By discussing the problems which each undoubtedly has, perhaps there will be more goodwill and a lot less misunderstanding.

Dentistry is practised by an honourable profession and as with all professions and organizations there may be a few black sheep, but these, although making headlines, are a very small minority. The extraordinary improvement in dental health, both child and adult, in the last few years is a testimony to the endeavours both in practice and research of those involved in dentistry today.

January 1985

Acknowledgements

My thanks are due to Dr A.H. Rowe, Professor of Dentistry, Guy's Hospital, London, for his advice on reading the text, and to the following for permission to adapt illustrations:

Dr H. Colin Davis, O.B.E. and
Miss Doreen Land, (*The Lecturer's Guide to the Mouth*)
Messrs Colgate Palmolive, Ltd
Dr John Chipping (*Your Teeth*)

1

The Goal: Beautiful Teeth and a Healthy Mouth

Most of us are born with the potential for a healthy body, a healthy mouth and attractive teeth. The faults which develop and show up in our teeth and jaws are rarely due to bad luck, but are mainly due to neglect or misuse by us or those around us. A small proportion of the population does inherit disfiguring mal-formations or acquires some diseases at birth, which can require years of treatment to put right. The possession of a set of healthy and beautiful teeth can contribute so much to personal well-being and satisfaction and we now know so much about how we can keep them for our lifetime, that it becomes a matter of wonder that we allow avoidable diseases to destroy one of our greatest personal assets and bring about changes in our appearance which can make us miserable. Nevertheless modern dental experts can work miracles in rebuilding broken-down teeth and jaws and the skilled dental surgeon and his team can bring about changes which not only repair the damage but can improve

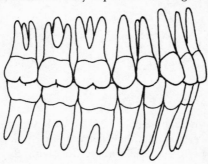

Figure 1.

11

their appearance and that of their owner almost out of all recognition.

In the diagram (Fig. 1) we can examine a perfect set of teeth in which the upper and lower teeth meet in a regular manner – not edge to edge, but overlapping like a closed pair of scissors. The teeth, in this way, function as a perfect cutting and grinding machine and they also look good. But the influence of regular teeth is far greater. Look at the lips and cheeks of a person with good teeth (Fig. 2). See how smooth and regular the surface of the skin is and how free from deep wrinkles. The teeth keep the shape and the muscle tone of the face. The next diagram (Fig. 3) shows features without teeth and the difference is obvious. The real age does not matter. Without teeth the chin gets nearer the nose and the face gets shorter, deep lines develop, and many years are added to the real age. If some good dentures were placed in this mouth in time most of the facial changes would be eliminated and the appearance improved.

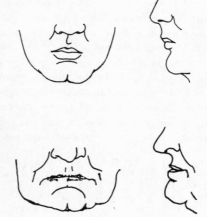

Figure 2.

Figure 3.

If we are fortunate enough to be born with the potential for good teeth we can preserve them by keeping to a few rules for their health and preservation. Incidentally, following the rules for good dental health will also benefit the rest of the body.

The dentist can repair or fill in any gaps caused by lost teeth, or crown any unsightly ones, thereby covering them with a better looking surface, usually made of porcelain. Treatment of this sort may vary from a few fillings to a complete dental reconstruction of all the remaining teeth. Such work can be very expensive. Because of the sophisticated and intricate materials and techniques involved *good dentistry* must be costly. But the *best dentistry,* which is *prevention* of disease, is quite inexpensive and so we should not, if we care, be considering any other course but prevention.

All the teeth can be extracted and replaced by complete upper and lower artificial dentures. There are dentists who are experts in making full dentures for those without their own teeth and the final appearance can be so good that no one would ever know that they were not a natural endowment. However, no expert in these matters can promise that more than a small percentage of his dentures can function, i.e. chew, stay in place and remain free from irritation, anything like as well as natural teeth. And there are some unfortunates who have the most beautiful and natural looking dentures but cannot get used to them. Just as some people can wear contact lenses and forget they have them in, usually after much perseverance, but others give up, so a similar attitude can be seen among denture wearers. The moral therefore is: however beautiful your friend's dentures may be and however happy he or she may swear they are with them, the result may not be the same with you.

So, beautiful teeth are best if they are natural, and even better if they have been so well preserved by preventive methods that very little repair work need be done on them. It is also better for your pocket. In later sections we will deal with ways of overcoming jaw defects and other problems which were caused by faults in the growth process.

For the moment, remember, toothpastes, although they have a valuable place in the hygiene of the mouth, will not make your teeth beautiful if they were not beautiful before you bought that tube, and there is nothing you can buy in the stores that will make them so. If you want to change the appearance of your teeth, the only one who can advise you is your dentist.

2
What You Should Know about Your Teeth and Jaws

The mouth

Explore your own mouth using your tongue as a guide. Lift up your tongue and feel it touch the flat rather ticklish roof which is the *hard palate* extending from behind the top teeth. This has a thin covering of tissue called the mucous membrane and has a sheet of bone underneath and divides the mouth from the nasal cavity above it. Going backwards along the hard palate towards the throat your tongue should just about manage to get to the *soft palate* which is moveable because it has no bone underneath. It hangs down rather like a curtain and has a protective action to prevent unwanted objects from being swallowed. Now bring the tip of your tongue towards the front again and touch your top teeth. The tip should be able to sweep around the arch of your top jaw and make contact with sixteen upper teeth. Similarly, your tongue can contact sixteen lower teeth – if you have them. These teeth are embedded in the jaw bone which is what holds them in place and this bone is protected by gum which covers it and, in a healthy state, prevents the entry of infection and undesirable intruders, just as the skin protects our whole body on the outside. The healthy gum around the teeth becomes quite hard and can stand up to the abrasions, stresses and forces created by chewing which could damage a softer area.

The tongue itself occupies a great deal of the space inside the lower arch of the teeth. Therefore there is no equivalent of the hard palate which we could feel between both sides of the upper jaw. The area in which the tongue sits is called the *floor of the mouth*. Under the tongue, buried in the floor, are glands which make

15

saliva, holes through which saliva is delivered, and numerous other glands, blood vessels and the tongue attachments, muscles for moving the jaw and tongue and other important structures. Therefore, although one can cover the top palate so that an artificial denture could rest across, this is not possible in the bottom jaw. Nothing could cover the floor of the mouth if only because the tongue needs plenty of room to move about. This makes the wearing of a complete lower denture much more difficult than an upper one because the former is confined to a narrow zone around the teeth, and the weight of it cannot be distributed over a large area for more comfort and balance (it's like riding a one-wheel cycle compared with a motor car). The lips and cheeks around the outside of the teeth are important and are made up of muscles which are concerned with chewing, changes in facial expression and various other functions.

The whole of the inside lining of the mouth (mucous membrane) should be of a light pink colour (called 'salmon pink' in the dentist's notes). The only red areas should be the lips and the inside of the lips where they join the gums. Any deviations from this, such as white or greyish patches or red areas, should be pointed out to the dentist when attending.

The teeth

Human beings develop two sets of teeth during their lifetime. There are twenty teeth in the first set (milk teeth or baby teeth). The second, the permanent set which replaces the baby teeth during childhood, numbers thirty-two teeth.

There are two jaws, upper and lower (the dental arches) which are each divided into right and left halves, making four quadrants (upper right and left, and lower right and left). Thus there are eight permanent teeth in each quadrant and they are numbered one to eight working backwards from the midline between the two front teeth. So the last tooth in the upper right quadrant is the upper right eight (the upper third right molar or wisdom tooth). The deciduous teeth are given letters A – E so the immediate front tooth in the four-year-old is A whilst the last tooth at the back is E.

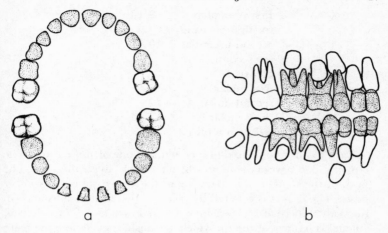

a   b

Figure 4. (a) shows the state of eruption of a child's teeth at about six years of age. The shaded teeth are the deciduous or 'milk' teeth. The four lighter teeth at the back of each jaw are the first permanent molars which erupt at about this age. In (b) we see the developing permanent teeth as an X-ray film would show them (unshaded here) buried in the jaws.

Primary Dentition – baby or deciduous teeth
NB: eruption dates for teeth vary widely

			average age of eruption (months)
A	=	central incisor	6
B	=	lateral incisor	8
C	=	canine	18
D	=	first molar	12
E	=	second molar	24

Secondary Dentition – permanent teeth

			average age of eruption (years)
1	=	central incisor	7
2	=	lateral incisor (or second incisor)	8
3	=	canine (in USA, cuspid)	9-11

4	=	first premolar (or first bicuspid)	9-10
5	=	second premolar (or second bicuspid)	10-11
6	=	first molar	6
7	=	second molar	12
8	=	third molar (wisdom tooth)	17-25

Each tooth is composed of a crown and one or more roots. The crown is that part of the tooth which is visible above the gum. The neck of the tooth is that part where the crown joins the root or roots. The crown is covered by *enamel* – the hardest substance in the body. There are no sensitive tissues in enamel. The colour of enamel is lightest at the tip which is translucent. Where the teeth are yellow this is usually because the enamel is thin and the more yellow dentine underneath shows through. The teeth themselves tend to darken with age.

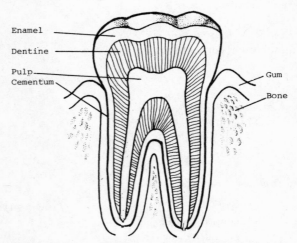

Figure 5. Section cut through a molar tooth and its support, showing the different structures.

Underneath the enamel and forming the bulk of the tooth is *the dentine* which is softer and less dense than the enamel. It is a sensitive tissue and therefore an *alive* tissue and, unlike the enamel, it extends into the roots. Inside the centre of the dentine is the *pulp chamber* which is a hollow cavity and is usually called the nerve. This is not strictly accurate because the chamber contains blood vessels, protective cells, nerve tissue and other materials necessary for repair. This pulp supplies sensation to the tooth.

The pulp chamber connects to the bone of the jaw through the *root canals* which are narrow pathways through which the nerve and blood vessels pass in and out of the tooth. The root itself is covered by a thin, hard, bone-like substance called *cementum* which stops at the neck of the tooth and does not cover the crown. It is perforated at the tip of the root (the apex) by the apical foramen (or opening) for the passage of the nerve and vessels entering the pulp.

The tooth root is joined to the bone surrounding it by a ligament (the *periodontal ligament*), which runs from the cementum to the

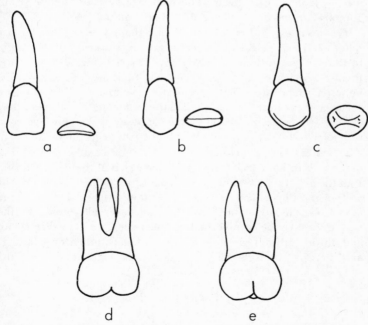

Figure 6. (a) incisor   (b) canine   (c) premolar
             (d) upper molar   (e) lower molar

bone. This ligament acts as a *shock absorber* and prevents the bone and tooth being damaged by a sudden excessive chewing or biting force. The front teeth (incisors and canines) all have single roots, the posterior teeth (premolars and molars) have from one to three or sometimes four roots.

The incisors at the front of the mouth have triangular- or spade-shaped crowns with usually sharp edges adapted for cutting the food. Place the tongue between the upper and lower incisors and *carefully* and *gently*(!) bite down just a little. It can be felt that it would not take too much effort to bite right through the tip of the tongue (see Fig. 6a). Place the tongue back between the molar teeth and start to close the jaws *gently*(!) a crushing action on the tongue can be felt, i.e. the tongue could be squashed rather than cut through.

The canines have pointed crowns which originally were meant for tearing food such as meat. The teeth are very prominent in all animals like the dog – hence the name 'canine' (see Fig. 6b).

Premolars and molars are more box-shaped, the *premolars* are narrow *chewing* teeth and the *molars* are large *chewing* and grinding teeth usually with four or more *cusps*. The chewing surfaces of the molars are broad and the surface is built up of these cusps, between which are valleys or *fissures* (see Fig. 7). The chewing surfaces of the back teeth are called the *occlusal surfaces* because they occlude (meet) with those of the opposite jaw. (Fig. 6c is a premolar, 6d is an upper molar and 6e is a lower molar.)

When the jaws are closed the teeth should ideally meet so that they mesh in with each other, with the cusps of the molars fitting into the grooves or fissures in the opposing tooth (see Fig. 1). The arch of the upper teeth is larger than the lower so that when the jaws close the upper teeth overlap the lower all round. As the human (unlike the carnivorous animals) does not chew directly up and down, the jaws can slide sideways on each other for grinding, and there is provision for the cusps of the teeth to slide on the

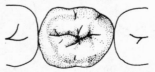

Figure 7. Chewing surface of molar showing crevices or fissures.

opposing cusp walls. It is important when dentists are restoring teeth for this delicate balance not to be disturbed.

Function

Teeth are necessary for: eating, speaking, appearance.

1. *Eating*. The teeth, tongue, lips and saliva all play a part in chewing. The lips first of all act as a testing area in order to reject food that is unlikely to be tolerated or could be harmful, e.g. too cold or too hot. Once the food is taken into the mouth, the lips close to seal off the liquid or food from being lost. The piece of food which was bitten off by the incisors and canines is then directed back by the tongue to the premolars and molars where it is crushed and minced up. The tongue also helps by crushing food against ridges in the palate and then, as it pushes against the roof of the mouth, forces the food into the throat in the action of swallowing. The tongue is important because the major taste organs are situated over its surface. They can detect salt, sweet, bitter, sour tastes; and all our subtle tastes are a mixture of these sensations. Thus the supposition that we taste with our palates ('He has a very sensitive palate') is on the whole incorrect, although there are a few taste buds in the palate. Of course the sense of smell is also important in the appreciation of food.

2. *Speaking*. If there are defects in the teeth or gaps caused by missing teeth, there may be mispronunciation of words, or sounds such as whistles or hissing noises. The positions of the tongue, palate, lips and teeth are important for good speech, and alteration in the relationship of these may need practice in order to compensate for the resulting sound changes. If there is a tongue-tie due to the tongue being too closely attached to the floor of the mouth by its string-like fold, there will be a tendency to lisp. This should be looked for early in a child before speech habits become difficult to change. The string can easily be snipped by a doctor without fuss or trouble, thus freeing the tongue.

3. *Appearance*. It is obvious that a pleasant facial appearance depends on the presence of all teeth (or nearly all), their position and the relationship of both jaws to each other (occlusion). If the upper projects over the lower too far with a rabbit-like appearance (called 'English teeth' outside England) the impression is usually one of weakness, i.e. with a receding chin. With a pronounced

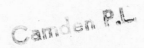

bulldog-like chin (the *Habsburg jaw*) the lower front teeth project in front of the uppers.

Elderly people who have been without teeth for a long time have a condition of *overclosure*. Here a great deal of bone shrinkage has taken place and it is almost possible for the point of the chin to touch the nose. Well-made dentures can often compensate for this loss of height.

3
Dental Diseases

In the main, dental decay occurs in youth and periodontal disease later in life. Dental decay is the more obvious to the public (and to dentists) because of holes or cavities in the teeth, and so most people think of dental disease in terms of tooth decay. However, the silent and usually painless periodontal disease is responsible for more tooth loss than dental decay and in spite of all the fillings that dentists insert, the populations of the 'civilized' nations still seem to lose their teeth at the same rate, because of progressive gum disease.

Dental caries

Dental decay attacks the enamel, gradually 'eating' in and destroying the inside of the tooth (the dentine). There are few people who have not suffered from dental decay at some time. If decay is neglected, the pulp inside the tooth eventually becomes inflamed, and pain is felt in various degrees.

Decay may not be visible to casual observation and may also not be painful until the 'nerve' is involved (dentists call this 'an exposed pulp') and thus regular examination is required to repair the defect before the dental pulp is reached. Once there is such involvement a simple filling will not suffice because the inflamed pulp usually needs special treatment such as root canal therapy (or the cleaning out and sealing of the nerve canal). Otherwise the drastic alternative may be the extraction of the tooth. (There are, of course, other alternatives but these will be discussed later in Chapter 14, Restoring Teeth.)

What is this thing called plaque?

Dentists will tell you about plaque and how it is responsible not only for decayed teeth (dental caries) but also for the inflammation of the gums leading to periodontal disease (pyorrhoea) and tooth

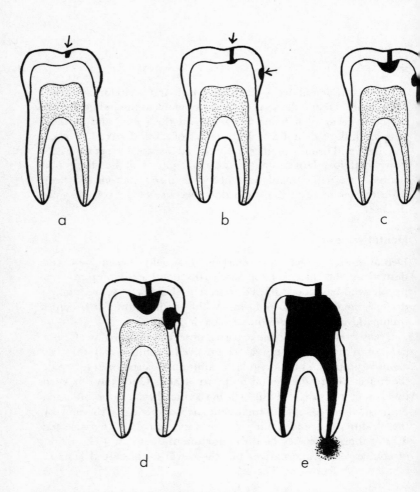

Figure 8. Progress of dental decay leading to abscess formation.

loss; you must learn how you can deal with it successfully yourself.

Plaque is not a new discovery. Hundreds of years ago it was known that if a film of dirt was regularly removed from the teeth the mouth was kept in good order. After all, the toothbrush was invented centuries ago expressly for the purpose of removing dirt and debris from around the teeth. But we now distinguish between food debris and film which forms on the teeth. Debris from food is looser and can be removed fairly easily, but the plaque film is more closely attached to the surface structure of the teeth. It is a sticky layer which is mainly made up of millions of bacteria and grows on the surface of the teeth and gums. It may be invisible or white, and therefore does not readily show up against the teeth. The most common place for it to accumulate is between the teeth and at the edges of the gums where they meet the teeth. The bacteria in the plaque make acid as they feed on the foodstuffs in the mouth, especially sugars, and this acid attacks the enamel, beginning the process of dental decay.

Other bacteria then go to work in the breached enamel surface and the decay spreads through the softer dentine under the enamel. The accumulation of plaque is made worse by sugars in the mouth, especially sucrose, and of course lack of brushing enables the plaque to build up on itself. The toxins made by the bacteria cause the edges of the gums to become inflamed and hence they enlarge slightly. This makes a ledge for a thicker film of plaque to collect and so a vicious circle is created. If this plaque is carefully brushed away regularly, the situation is reversed.

If the plaque is allowed to remain it hardens into calculus (tartar) which is not removable by brushing, but this deposit, because it is rough, collects more plaque on its surface causing further irritation.

The meaning of tooth pains

There are different degrees of pain connected with tooth decay and it is useful for the dentist to know the extent of the discomfort which has been experienced. It may have a great deal of bearing on the type of treatment to be given and the estimation of the future of the tooth.

1. A pain lasting for only a short time – a few seconds to about two minutes – brought on by food (often a sugary substance) getting into the cavity, or hot and cold drinks, usually indicates that there is a slight inflammation of the pulp which is reversible. That is, the pulp may recover if the dentist can attend to the cavity quickly, cleaning it out and possibly placing a sedative dressing in the deeper portions, and ultimately filling the cavity as soon as he thinks it is reasonable.

2. A longer lasting pain (say, twenty minutes) brought on by warm or cool foods or liquids is more likely to mean that the inflammation may not be reversible and the pulp may have to have special treatment.

3. Pain which seems to occur without any connection with food or drink and for no apparent reason, which is usually worse at night and may prevent sleep, is well-established pulpitis – inflammation of the pulp – and the dentist must be contacted right away. He will remove the pulp while the tooth is anaesthetized with a local injection or, in the extreme case where the tooth has so decayed that there is not much to rebuild, he will be forced to remove the tooth.

Thus, it is wise to take note of the early warnings, if there *is* an early occurrence of 'twinges'. There isn't always a warning – so we advise regular check-ups to detect trouble at the onset.

Some relief from continuous toothache can be obtained by taking two tablets of aspirin or paracetamol (acetaminophen) four-hourly. However, it probably will not work sufficiently. But one of the disadvantages of using painkillers to get over toothache and avoid seeing the dentist is that eventually the pain *will* go. This is no cure; what happens is that the diseased tooth is so damaged that the pulp dies. The trouble is that the owner of the tooth then feels a great sense of relief and may put off getting the attention needed. But a tooth with a dead pulp is likely to develop an abscess and, if acute, this is accompanied by pain and swelling and leads to much more likely loss of the tooth.

4. Thus we come to the next pain – an intense throbbing which may be experienced at any time of day or night, with the tooth being very tender to touch and perhaps extruded from its socket so that it contacts before the others when the teeth are brought together. The tooth may become loose and the sufferer becomes

hot and feels somewhat ill. This is the abscessed tooth mentioned above. In this state antibiotics may be necessary. If the abscess is large incision may be necessary to drain off the pus.

What causes dental decay?

We need not go into the various theories of the causation of dental decay, but it is generally accepted that dental caries is an infection, in that bacteria – micro-organisms – are involved. These feed on the sugars (mainly the sucrose which occurs in our sweets, biscuits, cookies, jams, chocolates, etc.). Acid is produced which dissolves the enamel, starting the decay process. There is no doubt that some people's teeth decay more readily than others even with the same consumption of sugars and the same brushing habits, and we know that one of the factors is the resistance of the tooth enamel to the action of the acid produced by the bacteria. This resistance may be something we inherit from our parents if we are lucky. We also know that the presence of traces of fluoride in the enamel surface makes it much more resistant to the acid attack.

Knock out just one of the factors contributing to dental decay and our decay rate goes right down. In the section on prevention we will explain just how we can achieve this.

The most likely parts of the tooth to decay are the areas which are difficult to clean thoroughly, either by the tongue or by the toothbrush. The biting surfaces of our back teeth have deep folds (called fissures) in them and bacteria and plaque can get down into the cracks making it difficult for the brush to get at them. Also, where adjacent teeth touch each other, sugary substances can cling to the area of contact and as this is difficult to brush out decay will tend to start here too. The dentist must investigate these hidden areas and often the only method to detect early decay in such places is to use X-rays with films specially designed for this purpose called 'bite wing radiographs'.

One of the main causes of decay is the eating of peppermint sweets (and other 'medical' candies). Many people believe that because of the peppermint taste there must be something antiseptic about these sweets. The truth is that they are especially harmful as they are often allowed to dissolve in contact with the side of the teeth. Dentists see enormous numbers of new cavities in those who have given up smoking and who compensate by sucking white mints. If you must have snacks, eat peanuts or crisps – they are less harmful to your teeth.

Gum disease

It was mentioned previously that all the fillings inserted do not prevent the majority of people over thirty-five from losing their teeth – because of progressive gum disease.

It is important to understand how the teeth are held firmly in the jaws.

The teeth roots are supported in the bone of the jaw but they are not glued to the bone immovably – there is a very slight space between the root and the bone all round and this is filled by a sling of fibres which attach the tooth to the bone. The spaces between the fibres are filled with fluid which increases the action of the fibres as shock absorbers and prevents too much jarring inside the jaws. Otherwise eating would not be comfortable. But, more important, the force of chewing or biting something hard would be directly transmitted to the tooth or its surrounding bone and one of these might be damaged every time we chewed something a bit too hard. The gums cover all the bone and are closely attached by the edges to the crowns of the teeth. This very close attachment helps prevent infection entering the bone area and thus also the rest of the body. Gum disease starts as:

1. *Gingivitis* which is the inflammation of the gums protecting the tooth support, bones and ligaments underneath.

2. If this is allowed to go on, the inflammation spreads because the gum separates from the teeth and allows the damaging infections to enter the pockets (space between the gums and teeth) so we have a deepening of the gingivitis.

3. The underlying bone holding the tooth is then progressively attacked and destroyed (*periodontitis*) and eventually, if enough bone is destroyed, the tooth will become loose and will be lost.

Remember, periodontal disease is not usually painful and therefore it is necessary to check regularly. The following are usually quoted as the warning signs of gum disease. If you answer 'Yes' to any *one* of these questions you should see your dentist and ask him to check your gums carefully.

A. Do your gums bleed when you brush your teeth?
B. Is your breath bad?
C. Are your gums soft, swollen or tender?
D. Is there a discharge (pus) from the gum line or in between the teeth when pressed?
E. Are the gums shrunken away from the teeth?
F. Is there any change in the way the teeth come together?
G. Are your front teeth starting to move, or space out?

Gum disease results from bacteria infecting the area around the teeth. Bacterial numbers increase very rapidly and, together with substances from the saliva, form the almost invisible film on the teeth called plaque. Calculus appears as a white or almost tooth-coloured deposit on the teeth along the gum line as the soft plaque becomes hard. Calculus can be found under the gums as they become inflamed and split away from the teeth. In this region it is usually black owing to the inclusion of colouring from the blood oozing from the inflamed gums. This calculus (tartar), like plaque, is made up of bacteria, mineral salts (calcium) and water. The tartar is built up in layers and, as it forms, each layer is covered with plaque and bacteria thus adding to the inflammation of the gums. Plaque also collects around those fillings which are not smooth or have broken edges. Thus the best way to prevent and minimize gum disease is to make sure you remove the plaque from both the gums and the teeth.

Remember more teeth are lost through gum disease than for any other reason. See your dentist if you have any doubts and make sure you emphasize your concern over your gums. A dentist should be able to diagnose any periodontal disease from the signs. The colour and shape of the gums is noted and the teeth are checked for looseness. Thin probes are gently and carefully inserted between the edges of the gum and tooth to measure the depth of any pockets. Nearly always X-ray films are taken to find out the extent of bone loss, if any, around the teeth. The way the teeth meet is also investigated in case the jaws have changed and some teeth are meeting unequally so that too much stress is being exerted on the bone supporting them. It is also important for the dentist to check for nervous habits such as clenching and grinding teeth, especially during sleep, because these can contribute to the breakdown of tooth support. This grinding is called *bruxism* by the dentist. It often also leads to painful jaw joints (just in front of the ears) especially in the morning after waking. The dentist may make something called a *bite guard* – a small plastic shield – to be worn at night to protect the jaws from the grinding effects.

Preventing gum disease

The best and really the *only* straightforward way is to make sure that plaque is removed from the teeth just as soon as it forms. As the amount of sugar you take increases, the amount of plaque also increases, and as sugar feeds the bacteria in the plaque, you should obviously cut down on sugary snacks and sweets, and remember that peppermint sweets are almost pure sugar. Cutting these down will reduce plaque and therefore gum disease and also reduce the incidence of tooth decay!

Plaque is removed by *effective* brushing (see page 66), and some people may have to use dental floss. You must be sure you are removing as much of this dental plaque as you can. Just brushing round your teeth haphazardly won't do. Plaque can be revealed by using harmless dyes. Effective dyes you can use are:

1. A food colouring matter – Erythrocin dye (in pink food dye FDC3 from food stores).
2. 'Displaque'– from your local chemist. In tablet (wafer) or liquid form.
3. Other dental disclosing solutions which your chemist stocks.
4. At a pinch you can use simple tincture of iodine, carefully applied to the teeth and gums.

Rinse once after applying these dyes and the plaque will show up clearly. Now make sure you remove as much as you possibly can.

Daily cleaning will keep the formation of plaque and calculus right down, *but* it will not remove it all because very few people are quite that perfect in their ability. So calculus which will form eventually in the mouths of most of us must be regularly removed by the dentist or the hygienist. Removal of calculus is called *scaling*. It is carefully and gently done, either by hand instruments and/or by use of an ultrasonic scaler which vibrates off the tartar after which the teeth are smoothed and polished. The dentist or hygienist will then advise how your own cleaning can be improved and may suggest a brush suitable for your mouth. However, the daily routine of plaque removal is up to you. Many patients tell us that they cannot understand why we make so much fuss about the plaque on their teeth. After all, they have always brushed their teeth three times a day, if not more. We have to point out that it is not the frequency but the success that matters. Brushing once a day would be sufficient if it removed all the bacterial film! You can buy a dozen sweepstake tickets – it's only the winning one that matters.

There are some general conditions which may exaggerate or worsen the inflammation brought about by the accumulation of plaque. Diabetes, even with adequate insulin injections, is difficult to control in its effects on the system. Diabetics therefore have to be especially careful about their mouth cleanliness. Similarly, *pregnancy* causes hormone changes in the blood and tissues and this can make an existing gum condition much worse. But a clean, plaque-free mouth in the pregnant woman does not become diseased.

So, the lesson we must bear in mind is that plaque is the main danger to the gums, not the systemic changes. In the same way, medicines which some people have to take will cause changes in the gums (enlargement). This can be seen in those taking certain drugs for epilepsy. But again it must be emphasized that if the mouth is kept really clean there is very little gum disease or enlargement.

Mouthbreathing where lip closure is inadequate (see Fig. 9) may cause inflamed gums because the drying effect leads to an insufficient flow of cleansing saliva.

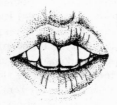

Figure 9. Inadequate lip closure leads to drying of the gums and may also allow the front teeth to drift forward.

Treatment of advanced gum disease

In the early stages treatment consists of thorough cleaning and curetting, (scraping away all the infected plaque and inflamed tissue in the pockets) and careful polishing. The inflamed gums will soon shrink and, with the help of scrupulous home cleaning there should be a great improvement. The thorough cleaning by the dentist or hygienist may take three or four visits, each time finding more tiny scraps of calculus that might not have been accessible under the previously inflamed gums. Each visit becomes easier for the patient and for the dentist and perhaps the gums in early stages of disease will return to normal. Careful maintenance, i.e. regular inspections, will be necessary to ensure no recurrence, and to see that the home care is being properly carried out.

All this may be done by your usual dentist, but often he will refer you to a specialist in gum disease and treatment, a *periodontist*.

In more advanced cases, and after all the calculus and plaque removal and home care, some deep pockets still remain in the gums. They can be eliminated by minor surgery under local anaesthetic. This operation is called a gingivectomy and is quite simple. The wound is covered with a dressing (a periodontal pack) which is left in place for about one week. Sometimes with even deeper loss of bone around the teeth a 'flap procedure' is done. The gum in the diseased area is lifted away from the teeth and all the diseased tissue and calculus underneath are removed and the bone may be reshaped. The gum is then replaced and sewn into position. This is done under local anaesthetic and is usually relatively comfortable while healing takes place.

Sometimes, if bone destruction around a back tooth is very severe and one of the roots of a three-rooted molar (in the top jaw) or two-rooted molar (in the bottom jaw) is hopelessly affected, it may be cut away from the rest of the tooth and removed, leaving the remaining one or two roots. These roots will then require removal of the dental pulp and insertion of a root filling to seal against infection. Such teeth may function very happily for many years. They often do not look any different.

Another advanced technique which periodontists carry out today is grafting new gum to replace a deficient area. The small graft is usually taken from another part of the mouth from which it can be spared, often the palate. The area from which the graft is taken, the 'donor' area, heals remarkably quickly. Similarly in some cases bone grafts, taken from another part of the jaw (only tiny amounts are necessary), may be used to fill in bone which has been lost from around a tooth.

But this is not the common run of gum treatment. The usual pattern is as we have described earlier – scaling, cleaning, cleaning and cleaning(!) by the dentist or hygienist and by you. This is where the remarkable improvement takes place. If the patient does not carry out the minimum home care required of him, the dentist is usually not prepared to persevere because an important part of his treatment plan will be missing. Everyone who is thinking about having crowns, bridges or cosmetic dentistry of any sort should be careful to see that the gums are in perfect order and that their plaque control is good. Otherwise the gums may shrink back to health one day – after the crowns have been made – and the edges of the crowns will be unsightly (see Fig. 10). If the gums don't shrink back you are in a mess anyway because eventually the pockets will deepen and the teeth with the expensive crowns will get loose. You can win only one way – keep your gums healthy.

If you have had periodontal disease which has been successfully treated, it is important to realize that it is not like having your tonsils out and then forgetting it. Periodontal disease can be checked and its ravages controlled but there will always be the need for vigilance. It calls for regular visits to the dentist or periodontist and careful following of the prescribed home care routine.

There is one particular type of acute gum disease which does cause pain and sometimes there is a fever and the patient feels ill.

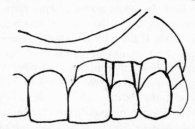

Figure 10. Unsightly appearance of crowned teeth after gum recession.

This is an infection called *Acute Ulcerative Gingivitis* (in the USA: Necrotizing Ulcerative Gingivitis, NUG), or Vincent's infection or, in the First World War, 'Trench Mouth'. This infection is more common in young people in their late teens and early twenties and may be associated with erupting wisdom teeth which have become infected. The gum points (papillae) between the teeth are destroyed leaving punched out gum craters which collect bacteria and dead cells. The whole area is very sore and is covered by a greyish white area of dead tissue. The breath is foul and there may be increased saliva. It is almost an invariable fact that the sufferer is a heavy smoker, and may also be a worrier!

For treatment you should see the dentist at once, and try to stop smoking and worrying. In the meantime a mouthwash of 10 volume hydrogen peroxide diluted one to three in warm water used three times a day should help. But if expert advice is obtained quickly and treatment is conservative the gums may return almost to normal, providing careful cleansing is performed at home. The dentist may put the patient on a drug called Flagyl (metranidazole) at the beginning of treatment. This is effective in about two days and the mouth feels comfortable again. The danger then is that the patient does not return for the most important part of the treatment, the cleaning and removal of plaque, calculus, etc. It must be emphasized that those who have suffered from Acute Ulcerative Gingivitis (AUG) will find the infection recurring unless they are very careful. Each recurrence will lose a little more gum with damage to the underlying bone and the teeth will become loose. To avoid recurrence it is essential to attend to the cause. The AUG victim is susceptible to *very small amounts* of plaque in the mouth, so for a long time, while this susceptibility lasts, great care must be taken about plaque removal. The dentist may advise attention to the other factors involved, such as partly erupted wisdom teeth. If they are constantly becoming infected he may recommend their removal. (This may be easy – not all wisdom teeth are difficult to remove.) Finally, remember that if you want to keep your teeth all your life the most important action you can take is to make sure that both you and your dentist pay careful attention to your gum condition. If you have the slightest doubt ask your dentist to refer you to a periodontist.

Gum treatment and the third-party paid services

One of the grave disadvantages of dental services paid for by insurance and other schemes (including the British National Health Service) is the poor provision made for treatment of anything more than the simplest gum disease. Specialist treatment for advanced periodontal disease is very difficult to obtain because of the still scarce distribution of periodontal specialists in any country. Some patients may be referred to dental teaching hospitals if they are accessible, but much of the work may be carried out by students and there is necessarily considerable delay before treatment is undertaken and perhaps a greater delay during treatment. With the growing awareness by dentists of the importance of periodontal disease in tooth loss it is regrettable that delays arise. Thus, for the majority who may not be able to afford to consult a periodontist, treatment is mostly confined to the simpler cases. Early treatment or preventive measures on the part of the dentist are essential and so is very careful home care on the part of the patient. Another stumbling block is the very low sums usually allocated for periodontal care by insurers throughout the world, which would discourage complicated treatment, while not quite encouraging extraction of the affected teeth. It does tend to bring about an attitude of 'Let's leave things alone until the teeth need to come out'.

The reason for the low fee scale may be the almost impossible task that third-party insurers have of checking the extent and the necessity for the provision of gum treatment.

Other diseases of the mouth

Diseases of the mouth may be acute or chronic. Acute diseases arise suddenly. They may be painful and may be accompanied by a general feeling of being unwell. If there are spots or blisters in the mouth or on the lips and these occur on other parts of the body at the same time, the family doctor should be consulted. It could be an infection such as measles or chicken-pox or other systemic infection.

A fairly common acute disease, especially occurring in infants is *herpetic stomatitis*. The mouth is very sore and the patient feels ill –

as in an attack of influenza. However, there are little blisters all over the inside of the mouth and palate and also on the lips. The tops of the blisters are soon lost leaving a raw (ulcerated) surface. Eating becomes difficult because of the pain. This is a virus disease and there is no specific drug used in the cure. The dentist may, however, prescribe aureomycin mouthwashes because they help to prevent the raw surfaces becoming infected by other bacteria and therefore promote healing and relieve pain. In any case, the condition resolves itself in about ten days. We usually say 'with treatment you will get better in ten days; without treatment it will take a week and a half', but the necessary general care is the intake of plenty of fluids and an attempt should be made (because of the aversion to eating) to get the patient to take nourishment – soups, soft food, etc. In general if eruptions or sores are confined to the area of the mouth it is probably better to consult your dentist first. If he considers the condition due to some systemic upset he will refer you to your doctor.

It would serve no useful purpose to describe here all the upsets which can occur in the mouth. The sensible approach should be to seek professional advice for any unusual change in the mouth which persists for more than a few days. Some people are subject to outbreaks of ulcers in the mouth. They may be single abrasions, sometimes under the tongue or inside the cheeks, and can occur singly or in crops. These are painful but usually quite harmless and heal after a few days, perhaps to return in another spot sometime later. Dentists call these *aphthous ulcers*. Although a great deal of research on them has been carried out over the years there is no evidence as to their causation. Treatment is therefore directed at easing discomfort. The dentist may refer persistent cases to a specialist in *oral medicine* for further diagnosis and treatment. All *persistent* ulcers or swellings should be seen by the dentist. It would be of assistance if a careful note is made of the approximate date of the appearance of the sore spot, whether it always occurs in the same place, or seems to re-appear elsewhere in the mouth.

White or grey patches may be noticed on the inner parts of the mouth, for example the cheeks or the tongue. Heavy smoking may cause some white patches and often these will disappear in time if smoking is given up. However, as before, advice should be sought in order to establish a correct diagnosis of the nature of the trouble.

Malignant mouth tumours

While most ulcers, swellings, etc., in the mouth are innocent, do not threaten life, and disappear in time, occasionally, as in other parts of the body, malignant tumours (cancers) can develop. These are rare, although it is probably true to say that fear of cancer (cancerphobia), without genuine foundation, gives unhappiness and distress to far more people than fear of other diseases.

In the UK and USA malignant growths of the mouth tissues are rare when compared to those occurring in other parts of the body such as the lung, breast, stomach, etc.

About 2,400 new cases of mouth cancers are registered annually in Britain, and lip cancers, which are the most common, are the easiest to treat if discovered early. It is hopeful to note that there is an eighty-three per cent five-year survival rate with early treated lip cancer. Another encouraging fact is that mouth cancer is diminishing in incidence and this is especially true in men. Whether or not the static rate in females is due to the increase in smoking among women in recent years is a question which requires further study. However, everyone should be aware of the following points: The evidence shows that there is a positive relationship between *pipe and cigar smoking* and mouth cancer. Therefore all those who have switched from cigarettes because of lung cancer statistics should be conscious of the alternative danger. But in spite of the changes some people have made in their smoking habits, overall figures show a decrease in pipe and cigar smoking and an increase in cigarette smoking. This may partly explain the reduction in mouth cancer.

Heavy drinking, especially of spirits, has been shown to be associated with mouth and throat cancer. This is particularly worrying in France where the number of deaths from mouth cancer is rising fast and is linked to the consumption of strong alcohol. Much of the alcohol in the high cancer areas in France is the crude pot-still type which is prohibited in many countries.

One may also speculate that a factor in the decrease in oral cancer is the improvement in oral hygiene. All dentists know that oral sepsis is less common than it was even twenty years ago.

Many cancer specialists, while not being able to provide statistical evidence, feel that this is the single most important factor in the reduction of oral cancer.

However, early diagnosis and treatment is still the paramount factor in reducing mortality.

The sensible attitude to mouth abnormalities

1. Stop worrying about cancer – the worry may kill you – the chance of getting mouth cancer is 1 in 25,000 so that in a city the size of Manchester there might be only eighteen cases reported in any year.

2. Most ulcers and sores turn out to be innocent.

3. Any ulcer which does not heal after a week or so should be investigated by your doctor or dentist. The same applies to any lump or swelling in the mouth or neck.

4. Persistent grey or white patches or thickenings should be investigated.

5. The dentist or specialist may want to carry out a biopsy. This means he will inject a local anaesthetic round the suspect area to numb it and remove a piece for examination in the laboratory. It is a perfectly routine procedure and does not mean that you have cancer. The elimination of the possibility of cancer being present is the first item doctors and dentists are taught in diagnosis. Therefore do not go into a panic if a biopsy is done. In the vast majority of cases the result is a happy one.

6. We learn from statistics that the chances of avoiding mouth cancer are very high if you abstain from heavy drinking, smoking (all types) and maintain a clean, healthy mouth.

7. So don't make your life miserable by worrying about remote possibilities.

4
Some Worries

Receding gums

Receding gums are not necessarily diseased gums. Nevertheless, a great deal of confusion and anguish has been experienced by many people of all ages when told by dentists that they have 'receding gums'.

If you have got this far in this book you should know that it is not the gums but the underlying bone of the jaw which grips and supports the teeth. The gums are important as a cover and protection for the underlying tissue, just as the skin and flesh protect the rest of the body. So what is most important in the preservation of the teeth is the amount of underlying bone.

In fact, in many of the bad cases of periodontal disease the gums are *enlarged,* covering more of the teeth than is normal, and careful examination by probing and X-rays reveal so much loss of holding bone that the teeth are loose and may require extraction. One of the ways in which a gum specialist may treat such cases (as we have already shown) is to remove this excess gum almost down to the level of the residual bone, so eliminating any pockets – gaps leading down from the edge of the gum to the level of the bone. Therefore such treated gum disease cases may have 'receded gums' but the condition may be quite healthy.

Some people become so worried about their receding gums that they come to believe they have a cancerous condition. Receding gums are often the result of a discrepancy between the size of the jaws and the teeth in them. It can sometimes be said that the patient has chosen the wrong parents, perhaps a father with large teeth and a mother with small jaws! We often find that the teeth are too large for the jaws, and the roots therefore are only thinly covered by bone. The gums in a healthy person fit tightly over the bone underneath – the mould of the bone actually determining the shape of the gums, just as the form of the hands and fingers will shape tight gloves. If the gloves are slightly too small for the fingers the tips of the fingers may eventually poke through until a state of equilibrium is reached. Similarly, if the teeth are large the gums are stretched too tightly over the necks of the teeth and eventually slip back (recede) to a position of equilibrium. After maximum growth has occurred (at about eighteen to twenty) there should be no further recession.

However, many cases of gum recession are caused by incorrect brushing with a hard bristle brush. The dentist will show how this can be avoided. Recession is often accompanied by some sensitivity of the teeth to hot, cold and sweet substances because a small amount of root surface, not protected by enamel, is exposed in the mouth. If the recession occurred gradually there is natural disappearance of the sensitivity. If, however, it persists and is worrying, the best remedy is a rinse which the dentist should be able to provide or prescribe and which contains a dilute solution of fluoride. The rinse, if used regularly, protects against decay and reduces the sensitivity. The dentist can also apply medicaments to the sensitive areas. It is possible to obtain relief by the use of special toothpastes (Denquel, Macleans dentifrice for sensitive teeth, Sensodyne, etc). If some recession areas look unsightly it is often possible to graft new gum on to those areas. Sometimes the dentist will discover that the cause of some localized recession is premature contact between one or two upper and lower teeth. A small adjustment to the biting surfaces of the teeth may cure the problem, as will a change in brushing method.

Remember, receding *bone support* of the teeth is likely to lead to the loss of teeth if allowed to continue. Receding *gums* may or may not be of similar significance.

Receding gums have never been a sign of cancer.

Halitosis (or bad breath)

Many people worry about bad breath, either their own or someone else's. The advertising media have made much of the social stigma arising from 'offensive breath', just as they have stigmatized all body odours so that eventually it seems that we shall all go around smelling uniformly like strawberries or rose gardens. If the deodorant manufacturers have their way we should never countenance the odour of the human body.

That being said, some breath odours can be unpleasant. This may indicate a dental problem but not necessarily. My own experience leads to the conclusion that bad breath is often the result of causes other than a dirty or diseased mouth. The odours may be caused by factors in the mouth or by changes arising in other parts of the body.

Local Factors. Direct mouth odours may be caused by decaying food particles on or between the teeth, a coated tongue covered by a growth of organisms, unclean dentures, a stale smell of tobacco, imbibed alcohol, gum disease – with an especially foul smell from acute ulcerative gingivitis – other ulcerative gum conditions, an abscessed tooth with the smell of pus dominant, and healing wounds after mouth surgery or extractions.

All these are understandable and can be dealt with. Thorough cleansing of all the teeth by brushing and attention to any dentures may improve conditions. Most people do not realize how thick a coating can develop on the tongue and this can be removed by careful brushing or scraping.

Although there are many proprietary mouthwashes on the market – all fairly expensive – one cannot be sure that any of them will succeed except by the flavouring in the mouthwash masking the odour for a few minutes, if at all.

Causes arising away from the mouth (extraneous factors)
Although most mouth odours do not arise in the mouth it is obviously a good policy to make sure that the mouth is clean. It is just as important to check on the nasal and throat passages – a head cold with infected nasal passages, acute sinusitis (often with a great deal of pus some of which drips down into the back of the throat) and other more chronic infections such as tonsillitis may give rise to the odours. Probably an infected tonsil region, even in adults, is a more common cause of bad breath than we have thought – even if tonsils have 'been removed'. Any stumps of tonsil tissue left can become inflamed and infected.

Many waste products broken down from food and drink are excreted through the lungs and this applies to alcoholic drinks as well as pungent foods – onions, garlic, etc. Hence the motorist's 'breathalyser' test which checks the alcoholic content exhaled from the lung. This demonstrates very clearly the futility of trying to mask the odours that do not arise in the mouth with mouthwashes or tablets. If the cause is recognized, e.g. alcoholic intake, or foods such as the more pungent cheeses (limburger, gorgonzola, etc.), the remedy is obvious but not always applied. Acceptance of odours varies with local custom. It is doubtful whether any inhabitant of a Mediterranean area would find the smell of garlic on the breath objectionable; in fact after a time the olfactory nerves would be 'immune' to it. These odours are therefore a matter of social acceptance or not.

Halitosis may occasionally be diagnostic of a diseased state somewhere in the body. Therefore, in the absence of a simple explanation for offensive mouth odours, see your dentist and perhaps also your doctor. I shall not embark on a list of all the possible diseases that can lead to halitosis. Diabetes is one and is often first detected by dentists; it may give rise to a sweet 'acetone' type of breath. Occasionally bad breath can be a problem which, in spite of careful examination and diagnostic aids, has no detectable cause and therefore sometimes no immediate cure. Quite a lot of dentists themselves suffer from this very problem.

It is worth repeating: no mouthwash, dentifrice, gargle, cachous or tablets can cure bad breath. Many of the mouthwashes can be harmful if used on a regular basis. The effect of mint sweets or throat pastilles and lozenges used as breath disguisers can be disastrous on the teeth, causing rapid decay. A mouthwash made up of a teaspoonful of salt in a cup of warm water is as effective, and safer, than most commercial preparations. Finally, smokers please note that it takes many days, probably weeks, before the 'soaked in' odour of stale tobacco is eliminated from the body. The sooner you give up smoking the closer your friends will become!

Painful jaw joints (temporomandibular joint syndrome)

There is now in the dental profession a much greater awareness of the need for diagnosis and treatment of problems related to the two jaw joints. Patients usually go first to the doctor complaining of pain or clicking of varying severity (sometimes very intense), usually on one side of the face and neck. This may be in the region of the temporomandibular joint (just in front of the ear) and may make eating painful and difficult.

Often the sufferer is unable to separate the jaws, i.e. open the mouth, wide enough to insert the usual mouthful of food and finds it necessary to cut the food into smaller portions. The confusion which may arise in diagnosis and hence in treatment is due to the fact that pain is not restricted to the area of the joint but may be referred to almost any part of the head and neck. Thus, there may be constant or repeated headaches, clicking, 'neuralgia', apparent attacks of migraine or even the semblance of toothache. Neck pains from the jaw joints can lead to the diagnosis of vertebral disc troubles. It has been said that many patients, because of lack of diagnosis of jaw joint problems (dentists call this the 'TMJ problem' or otherwise 'pain dysfunction syndrome'), have been forced to dose themselves continually with painkilling medications and are sometimes led to consult psychiatrists; some learn to live

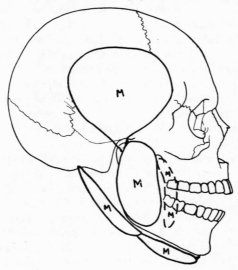

Figure 11. This shows some of the muscles of the jaws which need to coordinate.

with the pain because 'nothing can be done'. Others may have been examined for suspected brain tumours and even had major surgery to correct some other suspected cause.

The jaws are controlled in opening and closing and are maintained in position by a very fine balance between many muscles and ligaments which act together, some muscles contracting and others expanding in various movements of the jaws. Sometimes, because of interference to the normal movement of the jaws (perhaps teeth contacting unusually, or perhaps a poorly fitting denture), the lower jaw deviates slightly to avoid this interference, the muscles are thrown out of balance and, if this is repeated often, one or more muscles may go into spasm (like cramp in a leg muscle) giving rise to severe pain.

It is unlikely that the sufferer is aware of the interferences which start off the spasm. Of course, the total explanation is not simple, but once TMJ pain is diagnosed the pain can often be quickly, and apparently miraculously, relieved by discovering and eliminating the interferences. If the meshing of the teeth is at fault, careful grinding of the correct areas will achieve the required result. The dentist will take impressions and make models of the jaws to find out which tiny areas of tooth to grind. He may make a small appliance in plastic called a 'bite plane' or bite guard. This is usually worn at night and sometimes during the day as well. The bite plane has the effect of disengaging the interfering contacts and allows the muscles to relax. Pain therefore disappears if the trouble is indeed a TMJ problem and has been treated correctly. Even odd symptoms such as tinnitus (ringing in the ears), dizziness and headaches have responded to such treatment.

It must be stressed that TMJ syndrome is not the only cause of pain and problems in the head and neck. It has been assumed here that the possibility of dental causes, e.g. decay, abscesses, impacted wisdom teeth has been eliminated. If it has, and if the diagnosis does not point to the jaw joint and its musculature as the cause of the pain, full investigation, using all diagnostic aids, should be carried out. In this respect the panoramic dental X-ray is an invaluable aid and should be one of the first measures used.

How common is this problem? Some dentists may see approximately two such cases each week. Most of these patients have had pain for many weeks or months and in nearly all cases if the cause is as described above – pain dysfunction syndrome – there is usually relief in about a week or less.

It would be unfair to expect every dentist in general practice to be able to deal with a problem like this, but he may refer the sufferer to a specialist in a dental hospital for an expert opinion. The patient usually first visits his doctor with a complaint of this kind but in fact expert dental advice should be obtained as soon as possible.

Dry mouth (xerostomia)

There is a distinction between being thirsty and having a dry mouth. Occasionally continual thirst may be the result of disease, i.e. diabetes. But the continually dry mouth, which can be a distressing condition, is due to the absence or diminution in the supply of saliva which is produced from three principal salivary glands on each side of the mouth. The most noticeable effect of this lack of saliva, apart from the uncomfortable feeling of dryness, is the difficulty in swallowing food. With advancing age there is a natural slowing down in the activity of all glands and those making saliva are no exception.

In normal circumstances the salivary glands produce copious amounts of saliva which has a number of important properties:

(1) The digestion of some foods commences in the mouth by its contained chemicals.

(2) It lubricates food so that it can be swallowed easily.

(3) It has a cleaning action as a result of the almost continuous flow. (At night when flow is diminished there is always a degree of stagnation.)

(4) It has a buffering, i.e. neutralizing, action on many acids present.

(5) The tissues of the mouth are protected by specific substances dissolved in the saliva.

Thus an absence, or diminution, in the flow of saliva can lead to a large number of problems – a tendency for the surface of the mouth to become infected, difficulty in keeping the mouth and teeth clean and hence the possibility of rampant dental decay and gum disease. Because of the lack of lubrication the wearing of dentures is difficult.

We have all experienced dry mouth for short periods caused by emotional upsets – noticeably fear. Those suffering from depression may suffer from dry mouth, and at the same time the medicines and drugs used in the treatment of depression can have a marked effect in inhibiting the flow of saliva. A few sufferers from rheumatoid arthritis also have diminished flow. Intense radiation, used in the treatment of some disorders of the regions of the face, will affect the working of the salivary glands.

What can be done for this complaint? In the case of any persistent dryness, seek medical or dental advice, and there may be possible referral to a hospital consultant. A careful investigation may track down the cause which could be a medicine prescribed for another ailment. Many people with dry mouth suck acid sweets to promote the flow of saliva and also drink highly-flavoured soft drinks. Thus there is a risk of a high decay rate of the teeth. The dentist should be consulted so that he can advise on stricter oral hygiene measures and perhaps prescribe fluoride rinses.

The extent of the problem can be gathered from the fact that much research continues into the production of a harmless synthetic saliva. A reasonable amount of relief has been obtained by many patients using artificial saliva made up of a jelly-like substance – carboxymethylcellulose in solution and used frequently as a mouth rinse.

But remember, if you sleep with your mouth open or lips apart your mouth will feel dry when you wake up. This is not the same as dry mouth. However, your dentist may want to do something about this mouth breathing because it can make your gums inflamed.

5
Myths and Old Wives' Tales

It is strange how the teeth seem to figure in myths and legends throughout history. They occupy some deep area of anxiety in our subconscious as well as causing many of us concern in our waking hours. People often have dreams in which the loss or damage of teeth occurs. There seems to be a profound fear of tooth loss which, in more primitive times, arose from the difficulty in masticating food without teeth. In modern times the fear is probably more a cosmetic one.

Curious beliefs have originated over the ages because of the terror of toothache and the difficulty of dealing with the problem before anaesthetics. Countless types of toothache remedies were proposed and if the status of the advisor was that of a respected member of the community, the remedy was accepted as absolutely reliable. Unfortunately some of these remedies coincided with a belief (still existing among some primitive peoples) in the curative properties of urine, a 'universal panacea.' Perhaps it is an error to speak of primitive peoples because one cannot describe the recent head of state of an Asian country as primitive and yet he daily drank a glass of his own urine. In ancient times the first urine of the morning was advocated as a mouth rinse. Pliny (79–23 BC) recommended the toothache sufferer to, 'bite on a piece of wood struck by lightning' or take 'the juice of plants which are grown inside human skulls'. Ancient Chinese writings even alleged (fortunately for some, incorrectly) that tooth decay was advanced by excessive sexual indulgence.

The most common belief through the ages has been that dental decay was caused by worms boring into the teeth and eating away the inside. Dental decay, like gum disease, is caused by microscopic bacteria, and the breakdown of the hard tooth is started by acids formed by the bacteria from sugary food matter left around the teeth. This has been explained more fully in the section dealing with dental decay. Let us then list some current beliefs and deal with them as we go along.

1. *'Every pregnancy means a tooth is lost.'*

This is quite untrue and there is no reason for teeth to be lost if they are cared for. The belief could be based on the fact that a mother may care less for her mouth during pregnancy, and immediately after, because of other more immediate matters needing attention. This is discussed in detail in Chapter 13, The Mother and Child.

2. *'Whisky held in the mouth will help to relieve toothache.'*

Toothaches, which are generally an indication that the pulp of the tooth is inflamed, are sometimes eased by cold, sometimes made worse by it. If cold helps, whisky probably will too, by the cooling action of its alcohol. But it is probably better to swallow the whisky – if you like whisky.

3. *'Black people nearly all have marvellous teeth.'*

Because of the contrast with the skin colour, the teeth of dark-skinned people seem to be much whiter than those of European race. In fact, the teeth of black people may be quite yellow but look good because they are often slightly more pronounced and somewhat larger. The teeth of black people living in a primitive tribal state untouched by 'civilization' are usually very healthy. However, black people in cities have worse teeth on average than their white counterparts. This is related to the poor economic conditions usually encountered by recent immigrants.

4. *'It doesn't matter about saving the baby (first) teeth. They are going to be lost anyway.'*

If the first teeth are not cared for the following problems may occur:

    i. Decay and toothache necessitating extractions. This is a poor introduction to the dentist and to dentistry.

    ii. The first teeth help to maintain the place for the permanent teeth. If a baby tooth is lost early, the space may close up and lead to the permanent tooth being crowded out of position, making for a crooked row of teeth.

iii. If a first tooth becomes infected it might affect the growing tooth underneath and damage it.

iv. Taking a child to the dentist early, before there is any pain or discomfort (from two and a half to three years), will enable the child to have confidence in dentistry and make a friend of the dentist or hygienist. Prevention is much better than repair.

5. *'We all need glucose for energy and children therefore need sweets because they use up so much energy.'*
Most sweets contain sugar in the form of sucrose. This is harmful to the teeth and is not a body requirement for nutrition, energy or anything else. All the glucose you need is made in the body system from the normal diet. Extra glucose will be turned into starch or fat.

6. *'You've got to have false teeth anyway. Why not get it over and done with while you're young enough to get used to it?'*
This is a difficult statement to refute. After all, young men who lose both legs can manage to play golf and tennis. If this happens at sixty or seventy perhaps it is a wheelchair for life. The fallacy? You don't *have* to lose your legs – or your teeth. If accidents happen you have to make the best of it.

7. *'You can have new teeth screwed into the gums. It's the latest thing in America. Will you make me some? A friend of a friend had it done.'*
Dentists have been asked this question for generations. They may reply: 'Bring in your friend of a friend and if what you say is true I will do the same thing for you for nothing.' So far the challenge has not been met. Usually there has been a misunderstanding and the true picture is that the friend had all her teeth removed and new teeth fitted on a *removable* dental plate, but with the tips of the teeth protruding into the gums. Although this may look like a good thing to do, in general and in the long run, the teeth which stick into the gum delay healing of the jaws. Another mistake is to confuse the idea with post crowns where there is a root already present and a crown is fitted to it (see page 129).

There are of course such things as implants of metal into the jaws (or sometimes carbon implants). In the view of many dental experts these must still be considered experimental.

New teeth cannot be screwed into the gums. The best things to be buried in the gums and jawbone are your own teeth. Even a slightly loose tooth, if it is treated properly, is better than an implant (see Implants, p. 166).

8. *'All kinds of chronic illnesses like rheumatism can be caused by bad teeth – taking them all out will cure many vague diseases.'*
The theory of 'focal infection' where it was thought that an infected tooth could be the basis for much generalized ill health was responsible in the 'bad old days' for wholesale mass extraction and the fitting of millions of dentures. Unfortunately there are still a number of doctors who, if they are not sure what is causing their patient's illness, plump for 'bad teeth'. Apart from some rare exceptions this theory has been exploded and better diagnostic methods have established the reasons for the hitherto unexplained illnesses. The cause is unlikely to be 'bad teeth'. Taking out teeth to cure illness usually results in the patient with no teeth and the same illness.

9. *'Scaling damages the teeth because it takes the enamel off'.*
Scaling removes the tartar deposits on the teeth. Tartar may look like enamel but it is really hardened bacteria and 'dirt'. The main cause of tooth loss in adults is that these harmful deposits are not removed often enough, because some patients do not attend regularly, and sometimes not thoroughly enough, because it may require specialist attention. Enamel is one of the hardest substances known to man. It is very difficult to remove: if the dentist needs to remove it to make a crown he usually has to grind it off with *diamond* drills!

10. *'Fluorides are poison.'*
So are most necessary minerals and vitamins, if taken in excess. (But see page 62 on the subject.)

11. *'Fluorides are miracle medicines.'*
No. They are just basic requirements like vitamins. (Again, see page 62).

12. *'Clasps (wires to hold partial dentures in place) will rot your teeth.'*
A badly designed chair might give you backache. A well designed clasp cannot in itself cause dental decay or gum disease. However, it can offer a place where bacterial plaque can collect if the clasps are not cleaned regularly and thoroughly. Thus, clean clasps like clean teeth are usually safe.

13. *'Blackcurrant drinks are good for your children's teeth.'*
Many blackcurrant drinks like many other soft drinks are loaded
with sugar. They are therefore potentially harmful if the liquid is
left around the teeth. The reason for recommending blackcurrant
drinks is for the Vitamin C content. There may be better ways of
getting Vitamin C in fruit and vegetables. But a good rinsing with
plain water after a blackcurrant drink is a great help. Never, never
put these sugary liquids into baby bottle feeders or 'comforters'. A
normal diet should supply all the vitamins that are required; in
general *extra* vitamins are not necessary.

14. *'You are born to have good teeth or bad teeth and there is
nothing you can do about it.'*
A few people do have a congenital or hereditary disposition to poor
dental conditions. But these are rare and, on the whole, the future
of one's teeth is first of all in the hands of one's parents, then one's
dentist, if attended regularly, and – most important – oneself.
'Caring means keeping.'

15. *'I know sweets and chocolates and sugars cause decay so I
never have them. I give my children lots of honey and natural
sugars.'*
I have seen just as many teeth destroyed by 'natural sugars', e.g.
honey, being left in baby's feeding bottle for overnight feeds as
anything else. Most commercial honey contains sucrose which is
implicated in all dental decay studies. Substitution of one sweet
thing for another, even if it turned out to be less harmful, is not
good policy because you are still giving the child a sweet taste and
hence permanent desire for sweet food.

What is frustrating about all the above explanations is that in
spite of them many people will still go on believing the myths. I
remember one young mother coming to see me at the hospital with
a tiny baby whose mouth was in a dreadful state. I asked how she
cleaned the feeding bottles and she said, 'I rinse them in used tea
leaves.' I asked, 'You go to the child welfare clinic don't you? Did
they advise you to use old tea leaves?' 'Oh no. They told me to use
sterilizing solution, but my friend said old tea leaves were better.'

6
Home Remedies

Toothache

If toothache occurs the best course is to see a dentist. When you telephone it is important to make it quite clear you are in *pain* and are not just asking for a general appointment. It has often been found that patients do not state firmly that they are in pain and that an urgent visit is necessary. No dentist, however busy, will refuse to help someone in pain even if only to place a sedative dressing until a proper time can be found for whatever requires to be done. During the night or until the visit to the dentist, take pain relievers such as paracetamol (acetominophen) or aspirin. If you can see a definite hole in the tooth which is troubling you, a *small* ball of cotton wool (about the size of an orange pip) dipped in oil of cloves, squeezed almost dry and placed in the hole, should help. Failing oil of cloves, you can use oil of wintergreen, or even oil of eucalyptus. *What you must not do* is put any of these things on the *gum* around the tooth. Most important, *never* place an aspirin tablet on the gum beside the aching tooth. It will do severe damage to your mouth – an aspirin burn can be very nasty. Alcohol in the form of whisky is tricky. If you take enough you will forget your pain, but if put on the outside of the tooth it will chill it. If that helps why not use cold water? It's better for the mouth and cheaper! On the whole, painkilling tablets are much more likely to help than other remedies.

If you have a severe throbbing pain and the tooth feels as though it is raised out of the socket and is loose, it is likely that you have an abscess on the tooth. You can take your usual painkillers and if you cannot get to a dentist immediately, your doctor can possibly help temporarily by prescribing some antibiotic tablets. However, before you resort to this, try using a mouthwash consisting of a teaspoonful of salt in half a tumbler of hot water. Hold each mouthful for about one minute and repeat the procedure two or three times a day. You may find that suddenly your gum will swell up showing that the abscess has come through the jawbone to the surface of the gum and just as suddenly the pain will cease. The dentist will treat the affected tooth either by extraction or by cleaning out the abscess through the root canal. By this time the pulp will be dead and so the treatment should be quite painless. The important thing is for the dentist to drain out the infected matter through the tooth so it does not 'blow up' again.

It is generally a waste of money to buy expensive mouthwashes or irrigating devices for syringing and washing. Warm or hot salt water is always as good as any expensive proprietary rinse (with a few special exceptions which will be dealt with later).

If you suspect an abscessed tooth (e.g. a continuous throbbing tender one) *never* put heat on the *outside* of your face, using such things as heated pads or hot water bottles. The effect of these would be to bring the swelling right out onto your face and the abscess might even burst through the skin and, who knows, might leave an ugly scar.

Sore and ulcerated gums

If your gums suddenly become sore and bleed very easily as they are touched and there is a bad metallic taste it is possible that you have developed acute ulcerative gingivitis, which used to be known as 'Trench mouth'. This is a serious gum disease, in that if it is not treated carefully and thoroughly by the dentist you can develop a chronic gum disease which can lead to periodontal disease (pyorrhoea) and eventual tooth loss. So get to a dentist as soon as you can.

What to do in the meantime

1. Stop smoking! Most sufferers from this disease are smokers, usually heavy smokers. So stop. If you cannot stop cut down to a minimum.

2. Use a hydrogen peroxide mouthwash. Keep a bottle of 10 volume hydrogen peroxide handy and dilute it in warm water one

part in three and use this as a regular mouthwash until the dentist can see you. Do not go on using hydrogen peroxide or other rinses of this sort (e.g. Bocasan) after you have started treatment. Your mouth may feel better but the trouble will not be cured until the dentist has given you a careful course of treatment. One other thing, and most important, try to clean your teeth, in spite of the soreness, gently but better than you have ever done before. This, more than anything – more than any mouthwash – will clear up the infection quickly.

Halitosis (bad breath)

No mouthwash you can buy will ever cure halitosis. The strong-smelling ones will mask your breath for a time and that is all. There are many reasons for halitosis and a few of them are due to mouth problems. Make sure that your brushing is carefully done and that you have missed no parts of your teeth. You might also try *brushing your tongue* because bacteria grow on the surface of that, too. The dentist will advise you whether your trouble is dental and it may be that your gum condition is such that pus is oozing out from under the gums. In that case thorough scaling and cleaning (it might take three or four visits) should either remedy the condition completely or go a long way to rectifying it. But, remember halitosis can come from infected tonsils, sinus trouble, catarrh and post-nasal drip, and foods you have eaten such as garlic, onions, etc. Or it might be caused by changes in your body metabolism. First get rid of the scum on your teeth and see the effect of that. If you don't believe you have scum (plaque) on your teeth get some disclosing tablets, use them and you will be astonished at what you can see. Sucking peppermints and other strongly flavoured sweets to mask the halitosis will ruin your teeth.

Loose fillings

If a filling, either a silver one or a gold inlay, falls out or is loose, and it happens sometimes, *do not* push it back in! This is the worst thing you can do. If the tooth is sensitive, rinse well and stuff the hole with a small piece of cotton wool or some temporary stopping if you have some, and get an appointment with your dentist. If the

tooth is not sensitive, leave it alone, but get that appointment fixed
up!

Loose crowns

Jacket crowns which are made of porcelain or plastic (the latter
may be temporary ones) may come loose and it will be
embarrassing for you to walk around with just a stump of a tooth
showing in the front of your mouth. One tip, which may help for a
short time until you get it recemented, is to scrape out carefully the
inside surface of the crown, wash and dry it and place a piece of
Kleenex tissue around the inside (yes, Kleenex tissue!). Push the
crown in place and with a little luck it will hold for a time. What
you *must not do* is to refix it with Araldite or any of the epoxy-glues.
These are toxic and may do you a lot of harm. Do not panic even if
the porcelain crown is fractured. Dentists all over the world keep
stocks of temporary spares and there is bound to be one near
enough in colour and shape to tide you over until a permanent one
is made. But, remember, do not accuse your dentist of negligence
if a porcelain crown fractures. They have to stand up to a great
deal of battering in the mouth and the wonder is that they last so
well. Other crowns are stuck into the nerveless roots of teeth on
posts or rods (post crowns) and these can be the bane of the life of
dentists. It is important that you do not stick this back yourself
even if you have a kind friend at home who has some dental
cement handy. It is possible that the post crown has come out
because the root underneath has split and a careful dentist will
always check for this before he cements such a crown back in place.
A split root under a recemented crown will soon blow up into a
severe abscess and swelling.

Dentures

If you break your dentures and try to glue them together with
adhesives you will find that this will rarely be successful. You may
also damage the denture so that the dental technician will have
difficulty in repairing it and new impressions and extra expense
will be involved. It is also dangerous, however desperate you are,
to take the denture to a denture repair shop. Many of the operators

of these establishments have little skill (unlike recognized dental technicians, overcharge enormously and may ruin your denture – some will try to persuade you to have a new denture which they will make (illegally) with the pretence that they will charge less than a qualified dentist. You stand the same chance as you would with some of the 'cowboy' plumbers who are operating today. If your denture is loose it may need a reline. This is a skilled task and calls for a careful examination of your mouth. If you are tempted to try the reline kits and materials that some chemists sell, you may not only damage the denture, but your mouth as well unless you are very careful. If such reline kits were any good, dentists would be using them too.

Chemists' remedies

Be very careful about using 'toothache drops', tinctures and other remedies. They may do more damage than good. If you have an abscess they will do no good; a hot salt rinse, holding the water in the mouth as long as possible, will do more good than most things you can buy. As with pain, before you can get to the dentist, one or two of your pain relievers – paracetamol (acetominophen) or aspirin – taken *four-hourly* should help a great deal.

The use of dental pastilles for a sore mouth should be looked upon as a very temporary help. Expert advice should be sought until the reason for the sores or ulcers has been ascertained.

A dental first aid kit

A dental care kit from chemists should include many of the articles below. Those purchased usually include toothbrush, paste, floss, disclosing tablets for plaque and a small dental mirror.

1. Small dental mouth mirror (ask your dentist or purchase one from larger chemists who have dental care kits).
2. Small packet of cotton wool.
3. Cotton buds (such as Q-Tips).
4. Dental floss – heavy, waxed.
5. Tweezers.
6. Small bottle of oil of cloves (about 5ml should be more than enough).

7. Small bottle of tincture of iodine (5ml).
8. Hand mirror.
9. Pen light.
10. Painkilling tablets, e.g. paracetamol (acetaminophen).
11. Small bottle of 10 volume hydrogen peroxide.

7

The Prevention of Dental Troubles

Much of this book would be unnecessary if dentists and the public followed all the rules of preventive dentistry. Dental decay (caries) and periodontal (gum) disease are among the most common diseases afflicting mankind, especially in the so-called advanced nations. The higher the standard of living, the more likely it is for tooth loss to occur.

As has been shown already, both dental caries and periodontal disease are the result of bacterial action in the mouth, in the *plaque* which collects on the teeth and gums. If it were possible to cleanse the mouth completely of the bacterial plaque and maintain it that way, there would be no decay and, apart from rare degenerative conditions, the gums would stay healthy. Thus we know what *should* be done – the difficulty is in carrying it out.

Preventive medicine has virtually eliminated many serious killer diseases such as smallpox, diphtheria, poliomyelitis and many others. The research facilities and worldwide public health measures were justified, whatever the cost, because of the lethal or severely disabling nature of widespread epidemic diseases. Dental diseases are not considered to be lethal and therefore attitudes on the part of governments and public are of a different nature. However, the cost of dental disease in pain, suffering, treatment and loss of work is enormous. Measures to reduce or eliminate dental problems would result in a vast benefit to the population. Fortunately, the last ten years has seen a tremendous surge in the demand for preventive care. Many dentists now believe in primary preventive care which means the elimination of the possible causes of dental decay and periodontal disease and helping the patient to practise all the requirements of home care.

Diet and dental health

The prevention of dental decay begins with cutting down the amount of sugars taken *in all forms*. Most people think we refer only to sweets as the culprits. But here is a short list of dangerous sugar-containing foods:

a. All sugars (including honey), even in tea and coffee.

b. Soft drinks such as colas and lemonades. Strong fruit juices, e.g. lemon juice, taken regularly will dissolve the enamel.

c. Nearly all cereals, even All Bran, contain large amounts of sugar. With sugar sprinkled on they are worse.

d. Cakes, biscuits and puddings.

e. Jam on your bread, marmalade on your toast.

f. Chocolates, sweets and toffees.

g. Peppermint sweets. These are the most dangerous because people believe the peppermint taste to be 'medicinal'. These sweets are almost pure sugar.

A popular chocolate candy bar of about two ounces may contain the equivalent of ten teaspoons of sugar! A slice of two-layer chocolate cake may be the equivalent of fifteen teaspoons of sugar!

These sugars are not an essential part of a normal diet so if we can reduce the total intake not only will the teeth benefit, but so will the general health. Nutritional experts like Professor John Yudkin believe that sugar in the diet is responsible for many of the ills of mankind. However, it is the *frequency* of sugar intake more than the total consumption which is important in influencing tooth decay. It was shown that the acid formed on the tooth in seconds from sugar may take twenty minutes or more to disappear from the mouth. Thus, small sugary snacks every two or three hours throughout the day will keep the teeth bathed in a dangerous acid state. Children, if they must have sweets, should have them at one period only of the day (preferably at meal time). But it is better to recommend sugar-free snacks. A good list would contain:

Fruits: apples, oranges, pears, bananas
Vegetables: carrots, celery, tomatoes, lettuce, cucumber, also nuts, crisps, cheese (in cubes), eggs, milk, yoghurt.

In Chapter 13, The Mother and Child, one of the early dangers is mentioned: the comforter or dummy dipped in sweetened substances and the small bottle feeder containing sugary liquids which can be kept in the mouth at bedtime and which causes gross destruction of the erupting teeth as well as developing a 'sweet tooth' for life.

If in this way we eliminate sugar, we reduce the formation of plaque and we deprive the bacteria of the food from which they form the acid.

Another way is to try to eliminate the bacteria. This is done by plaque removal as thoroughly as possible, by brushing, and also by the dentist treating already decayed teeth which are infected, but we hope that preventive methods will be adopted early so that decayed teeth are few or, preferably, there is no decay at all.

The bacterial plaque can be removed by brushing. Most people cannot brush *effectively* and should be taught to do this by the dentist, hygienist or other dental health educator. Children have difficulty in mastering toothbrushing until they are about seven or eight years of age.

Dental floss. Many dental health educators assert that even the most careful brushing does not remove all the harmful substances from the crevices between the teeth, parts where the bristles cannot reach. They recommend the use of dental floss, a special silk or nylon thread, which is passed into the space between the teeth with a *gentle* to and fro sawing motion. The floss is then gently worked up and down the tooth into the gum crevices. The floss is purchased wound in a spool and is either waxed or unwaxed. The vogue today is for unwaxed floss, but the waxed is easier to handle. Using floss is not easy and children especially have difficulty with it. It takes a dedicated and tireless parent to floss the children's teeth every day. It is far better to spend the effort on careful brushing.

Beware of the dangers of fruit juices taken immoderately as part of a slimming diet, for the complexion, or as a 'bowel medicine'. The damage by erosion which, say, lemon juice can do to the enamel has to be seen to be believed. So avoid too frequent tooth contact with lemons, grapefruit, vinegar and other strongly acid substances. (Ask your dentist – he uses dilute citric acid to etch the enamel for special filling techniques. It needs only to remain on the teeth for about *one minute* to eat into the surface!) The biggest proportion of victims are health food addicts, young girls and middle-aged people.

The chemist's shop may also be a source of danger to the teeth. Many cough and throat sweets, lozenges, syrups, and elixirs are loaded with sugar, sometimes up to 50–60 per cent. This is to make the product palatable.

Fluorides

A few dentists began using fluoride solutions as a preventive measure against dental decay over thirty years ago. This was by direct application, i.e. the regular painting of fluoride on the teeth of children from the age of two years. Since then the amount of decay in such treated children has been negligible compared with others. But it can be a time-consuming procedure although inexpensive compared with the cost and discomfort of dental decay. The addition of minute quantities of fluoride to the water supply, to bring the concentration up to the level found naturally in some waters, has been shown to confer resistance to dental decay.

Studies of the action of drinking water containing one part of fluoride in a million parts of water have been carried out in many countries in the world. Schemes to bring the concentration of fluoride-deficient waters up to the above level now function in thirty countries serving a population of about 150 million. Research work and enquiries have been instituted by such bodies as the Royal College of Physicians of London, the British Dental Association, American Medical Association, American Dental Association and many other responsible authorities in other countries. Because of the objections raised by various factions to the levelling up of fluoride in water supplies to the desirable level of one part per million (1 ppm or 1 mg per litre), enquiries such as that conducted by the Royal College of Physicians over a number of years have carefully examined the advantages and disadvantages of water fluoridation with particular attention to points of concern raised by opponents of fluoridation. These are the effect of fluoride on the skeleton (i.e. bone), kidney disorders, congenital malformations and cancer. The conclusion was that fluoride at a level of 1 mg per litre has been drunk for generations by millions of people throughout their lives. Since fluoridation was introduced millions more have been drinking water with fluoride at this level. In both situations medical and radiographic surveys have been carried out, sometimes covering areas with up to 8 mg of fluoride per litre. There is now an enormous body of information on the subject of fluoride and health which, the Royal College says, amply justifies the following conclusions:

1. Fluoride in water, added or naturally present, at a level of approximately 1 mg/litre over the years of tooth formation substantially reduces dental caries throughout life.

2. There is no evidence that the consumption of water containing approximately 1 mg/litre of fluoride in a temperate climate is associated with any harmful effect, irrespective of the hardness of the water.

3. In comparison with water fluoridation, systemic fluoride supplements such as tablets, drops and fluoridated salt have been shown to be less effective on a community basis.

4. There is no evidence that fluoridation has any harmful environmental effect.

In the absence of water fluoridation your dentist or hygienist can put fluoride directly on your child's teeth. This takes a few minutes and a strong recommendation is that it be applied at four-monthly intervals, i.e. three times a year.

Fluoride tablets and solutions can be obtained from your local chemist (see your dentist about prescribing the correct dosage) and these involve remembering to administer the correct amount daily, which may be a chore for some. But it is important to discuss all this with your dentist first. Some few complaints have been made about 'allergic reaction' to the fluoride tablet-administration. Investigations have rarely shown any true allergic response and any temporary upset has usually been due to other causes.

The dental hygienist

In Britain the dentists' increasingly favourable attitude to prevention is closely connected with the introduction of trained dental hygienists. Many European countries are starting dental hygienist school programmes and initially send their students to the USA and the UK for their training.

Dental hygienists entered practices hitherto devoted to repairing broken-down teeth and mouths. The effect of the dental hygienists' teaching was most profound on the dentists themselves.

The dental hygienist is therefore an asset to a dental practice. Do not take the view that she (sometimes he) is an inferior worker on whom you have been 'fobbed off'. The dental hygienist is an important member of the dental team and can usually carry out the jobs for which she was specially trained with a skill and attention to detail for which the busy dentist may not have time. She can carry out a large number of different tasks, among which are scaling, polishing, teaching home care of the mouth, giving advice on diet and nutrition, selecting the correct brush and dentifrice for the individual, teaching an effective brushing method, and if necessary, how to use floss or other cleaning items such as wood sticks. She can apply fluoride solutions, and (if the dentist considers these necessary) fissure sealants.

Choosing a toothbrush

Occasionally I stand at the toothbrush counter at chemist shops and watch people buy toothbrushes. Most of them hover over the shelves, picking up one brush then another. After some minutes they make a purchase, seemingly at random. When new patients are asked how they select a toothbrush, they usually say, 'Oh, I choose any brush really, one that looks nice in its wrapper.' A toothbrush is an important factor in preventing dental disease, especially gum problems. Therefore the purchaser should be quite specific when going into the shop. The dentist or hygienist will tell you which brush is suitable for you. Write it down and *ask for it*. Do not be fobbed off with something else 'almost the same' – try somewhere else!

Let us first of all dispose of the brushes we do not recommend. Expensive brushes are usually *not* satisfactory. These are probably hand-made (as if that made them better) and have natural bristles (hog bristles) or sometimes softer badger hair. None of these is satisfactory. Natural bristle was believed by many (dentists, too) to be better, but this is erroneous. Natural bristles have variable textures and the filaments are hollow and absorbent and rapidly become soggy and infected. Nylon can be made exactly to specification and, because of mass production methods, good brushes can be made much cheaper.

Brush heads should be small enough to reach all parts of the mouth and should have a flat brushing surface with a straight handle. The medium or medium soft nylon bristles (never hard) should be set close together – what is called multi-tufted. There is now a new British Standard (1979) BS5757 for toothbrushes and the well known makes conform to this. Brushes of any kind should not be expected to last very long and should be discarded as soon as the bristles splay out. The average adult should probably buy about four brushes per year. It is a sad fact that brush sales average about one brush per person per year with maximum sales during the summer holidays just before people go on vacation. Children need their brushes renewed more often as they tend to mishandle them. If an adult finds that brushes wear and splay out very quickly it is probably a sign that brushing is not being done correctly – probably force rather than care is being used. But some people are proud of wearing out their brushes: they feel they are doing a good scrubbing job!

Automatic (electric) toothbrushes

Many of the automatic toothbrushes produced a few years ago have now disappeared and there is no longer a great choice. The improved automatic brushes which are still available can be effective:

1. For handicapped people, especially arthritics.
2. For those who cannot master the technique of conventional brushing.
3. For those in a hurry and perhaps for those who are lazy.
4. For children who will often use the automatic brush more readily because of its novelty.

Nearly all automatic brushes have battery-driven motors and it is important to make sure that the battery is not in a run-down state, otherwise there will be too little torque (driving action) on the brush. Most of these brushes have rechargeable cells and they should be kept always at peak charge. People who can brush effectively with the usual brush will not need an automatic brush. It is still necessary to be taught how to use the latter; it will not go anywhere in the mouth unless it is directed. But the automatic brush does have the advantage of speed and that is why I prefer one myself, just as I prefer to use an electric shaver.

Cleaning the teeth

You cannot be taught to play tennis or golf by reading about them. You must be instructed, and you must practise. Similarly, if the dentist or hygienist sees how you brush your teeth he or she can correct any faults.

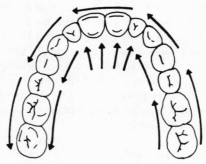

Figure 12. Systematic brushing of the teeth of each jaw. Each section arrowed requires about eight brush strokes. The arrows indicate the sequence of brushing each section of the mouth, not the action of the brush.

The back teeth have five surfaces – front, back, the two sides and the chewing surface. Brush the top and bottom teeth separately. Most dentists agree that the bristle tips should be applied at 45 degrees to the gum area just above where the teeth emerge and should concentrate on the gum margins (where most people miss). The bristles are moved back and forth with a gentle circular scrubbing motion and short strokes. Do not forget the teeth right at the back of the mouth and also the insides of the teeth. Finally brush all the biting surfaces. It often takes three or four visits to teach someone to brush effectively!

Notes on brushing. Do not put too much toothpaste on the brush, it will foam up and make you want to spit and rinse too soon. Our observations show that once people get to the spit and rinse stage they stop brushing even though some teeth have not been brushed. *Do not* wet your brush before applying the paste or before starting

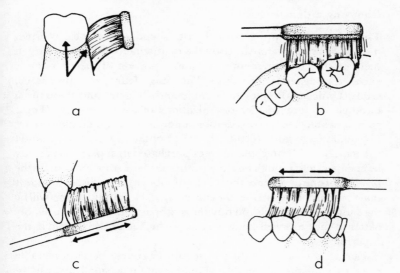

Figure 13. The sides of the bristles (a), not the tips, are applied to the gums and teeth and make full contact with all the curvature (b). The backs of the front teeth may be brushed as in (c). The biting and chewing surfaces are scrubbed (d).

to brush. It alters the action of the bristles and prevents them removing plaque effectively.

Using floss. This is difficult. Your dentist or hygienist must help you by seeing that you manipulate the floss correctly and safely. It is usually easier to handle the floss if a length of about twelve inches is tied in a circle. The best, easiest and safest material is called Dentotape made by Johnson & Johnson, and is sold in almost every country. Another excellent floss is called Super floss and resembles a pipe cleaner. Ask your dentist where you can get it.

Do not be seduced by special gadgets which purport to make flossing easier. None of these, in our view, does anything except add problems. What must be done is to get the strand of floss between the teeth, then wrap it partially round one of the teeth and gently sweep the tooth with it starting from the gum and ending at the biting surface. Do this sweeping motion two or three times and then repeat with the adjoining tooth.

Choosing a dentifrice

The big manufacturers of toothpaste spend a great deal of time, money and research facilities on the maintenance of high quality in their product. Their reputation, and a portion of their economic existence, depends on this. The 'big four' are Beechams, Gibbs/Unilever, Proctor & Gamble and Colgate, and there are a number of other smaller organizations of a similar type. These companies have spent considerable amounts testing their toothpastes and some have gone to the trouble of obtaining medical product licences. 'Own brand' toothpastes purchased in supermarkets may be cheaper, and though bearing the name of the store are usually the product of one or other of the 'big four' (above). One disadvantage is that you cannot be sure that the contents, or the manufacturer, will be the same the next time you buy the toothpaste, and so it is probably better to stick to a well-known brand – which may also be sold in the supermarket.

Pointers to choice. Toothpaste should of course be of acceptable taste to you and preferably should contain a small amount of fluoride. This has been shown to reduce dental decay by a measurable amount. On the whole it is better to buy small tubes rather than the large 'economy family size'. In this way the tendency for some pastes to harden in the tube will be avoided because the contents will be used quicker.

Other cleaning devices

Wood sticks and Interspace brushes. These are useful interdental cleaning devices, but do not use any of them unless your dentist has advised their use and has demonstrated them to you.

Water spray irrigation units (e.g. Waterpik). After testing gadgets which use pulsating water sprays and after considering the initial cost and the time and effort involved in their use, many dentists consider that they are of little value in removing plaque. The money and time would be better spent on more effective brushing.

The same criticism applies to *mouthwashes* and *gargles* used as a daily routine. Your dentist may advise a special mouthrinse for a short period for some specific condition. Otherwise there is nothing better or safer than warm water or warm water in which a little table salt has been dissolved (one teaspoon to a tumbler of water).

Fissure sealants. Decay frequently commences in the irregular fissures on the biting surfaces of the teeth, especially the molars. These fissures are difficult to clean thoroughly – a toothbrush bristle does not penetrate to the bottom of the fissure. In our practice we clean the teeth and apply fluoride, as already described. However, some dentists believe that these fissures can and should be sealed off from bacterial infection by the application of special resins which are made to flow into the crevices of the biting surfaces where they are hardened by chemical action or a special light. Usually at least the four first molars are so treated. But the fluoride applications must be used in addition. Again in our view, fissure sealants are rarely necessary as a routine and add to the cost of prevention without a commensurate benefit. But you must be advised by your dentist. His results may be better than ours, and fissure sealants are being improved all the time.

The future

Vaccination against dental decay?

I have explained how dental decay and most gum diseases are caused by infection by organisms. In most other infections we develop immunity after attack by the production of antibodies in our system. This is the basis of protection which we can give populations against diseases such as poliomyelitis, smallpox, etc. What happens is that a minute, harmless dose of the killed organism or its products is introduced into the body, which leads to the system interpreting the incident as a disease attack and it produces antibodies to protect itself against further attack.

Work has been taking place (and again the UK is in the forefront) in order to bring about immunity to the organism which causes dental decay. The work, which has been carried out on monkeys, has had encouraging results. These showed that unvaccinated monkeys fed on a diet containing sweets and sugary food developed decayed teeth while similarly fed vaccinated animals did not. It is hoped that, in the not too distant future, refinements in the vaccination materials, after much research and testing, may enable humans to be similarly immune to dental decay.

This research is full of promise. The brilliant workers in this field have already made many important discoveries and there are 'spin-offs' of knowledge even without the prospect of vaccination. As far as the medical prospects of vaccination against decay go it is easy to be enthusiastic. But we must take into account that dental decay is a non-lethal disease. Vaccination usually involves some risk (have not all vaccination projects had their disasters, however isolated?). One can understand the resistance on the part of some parents to whooping cough immunization, since there have been accidents with such inoculations. The effects of whooping cough can be much worse than dental decay. It would therefore be understandable if parents, however much they valued the teeth of their children, refused to take the remote risk of vaccination. We shall probably have the opportunity to make the choice within ten years. Perhaps dental decay will become of minimal importance.

8
About X-rays

X-rays have helped mankind greatly in the discovery, diagnosis and treatment of disease. Modern first-class dentistry is dependent for its success on careful X-ray examination, but there is a large number of people who fear that X-rays will cause damage. In fact dental X-rays today from modern machines with fast film are much safer and give a lower dose of radiation than that received from natural sources. There were cases of damage during the early days after the discovery of X-rays by Roentgen, because the operators and technicians were not aware then of the dangers of excessive repeated dosages. So most of the people who were harmed years ago were the radiographers and radiologists, not the patients. Today, with the knowledge we have and the advances in technique, dental X-ray (radiography) is quite safe for diagnostic purposes.

Thirty years ago the exposure for an upper front tooth was 5.5 seconds. The same X-ray is taken today in 0.3 seconds, which is about one-seventeenth of the previous exposure, owing to the improvement in film speed.

In dental X-ray examinations the rest of the body is often protected by the use of lead-lined aprons or shields. There are also diaphragms which reduce the spread of the X-rays from the head of the machine.

Advanced gum disease which has spread to the bony support of the teeth will be detected at an early, treatable stage if a complete X-ray examination of the jaws is carried out. There is no doubt that as far as dental health is concerned the patient will come to far more harm from neglecting to take regular X-rays than from radiation.

There are a number of different examinations the dentist can do for the patient. These are:

1. Complete mouth examination (about fourteen films are used). This may involve a total exposure time of about five to fifteen seconds. Such examination for those with a complete or almost complete set of teeth, should be taken at about three-yearly intervals, but of course your dentist may decide to shorten the period or, if there is no question of any dental health problem arising, the interval may be lengthened. The total procedure takes about fifteen to twenty minutes of chairside time. Added to this must be the time needed for developing and processing the film, mounting on card, etc. Then the dentist must take some time to examine the *mounted* radiographs and make a report on them. So such an examination cannot be inexpensive.

A few patients with sensitive mouths tend to gag or retch when a film – even a small one – is placed in the mouth for a short time while the exposure is being made. If the dentist sprays the back of the film – the side that touches the palate – with ethyl chloride (a cold spray) before he puts it in the mouth, the gagging is prevented. Very few dentists know about this, or if they do they do not believe in it; those who do try it are amazed that the simple remedy works.

2. Some dentists have invested in a very expensive *panoramic X-ray machine*. This scans around the head with a large film which is about 300mm x 150mm (12" x 6"). This film of course is not put in the mouth and the resultant exposure shows all the teeth plus many other structures of the jaws and face on one film. It is ideal for showing the developing teeth of children and the position of wisdom teeth. Although the detail of each tooth is not as fine as with a single X-ray film taken inside the mouth (the intra-oral film) the dosage of X-ray radiation of the panoramic film is very low and thus the technique, in which one can see both jaws and teeth arranged on one film in a few minutes, is a very useful aid.

3. *Bite wing radiographs*. In order to look for decay between neighbouring teeth where they contact each other, which is difficult to see in ordinary examination, two films are used, one on each side. These films are usually taken annually.

The safety of dental X-rays has been stressed here. Full safety depends on modern equipment and careful technique. The electronic timers, which are almost silent, are an improvement because they allow automatic accurate exposures to fractions of a second. There are special film holders for accuracy of angles, but there is no real objection to the patient holding the film in position. However, the dentist or his nurse should not hold the film in the mouth for you while the exposure is being made. They are dosing themselves continuously and unnecessarily. Many dental practices have regular checks by radiological safety organizations which ensure that the apparatus has been tested for safety. The operators may also wear monitor badges which record any stray radiation in the room. Finally, however safe dental X-rays may be, it is better to postpone radiographs for pregnant women until after childbirth. In emergency cases, essential dental radiographs during pregnancy can be taken with short exposures and with careful use of lead screens and aprons. Other patients who are concerned because they have had large doses of X-rays for other body examinations should discuss this with the dentist. To those who are anxious or fearful of the effects of X-rays, one could say that if the dentist uses modern equipment and takes X-rays when he thinks they are necessary, if the patient could live until the age of ninety then his or her life would be shortened by only one hour by the effects of the X-rays.

9
Accidents

Some accidents may be inevitable but others can be avoided and their effects minimized. For example, the use of seat belts in motor cars does not reduce the number of accidents but it does reduce the risk of injury or its severity. Similarly, in the known contact sports such as boxing, the use of mouth shields has made tooth breakage or loss a rare occurrence. It is in the activities where mouth protectors are not usually worn that we find most injuries. In children of school age the highest risks of tooth breakage and damage occur in: cycling; swimming; cricket; baseball; swings; fights and 'horseplay'.

Adults are less likely to be affected by sports accidents, but probably the most dangerous sport for teeth is squash racquets. Of course, a tremendous amount of damage is experienced by both children and adults in motor accidents and, as I've pointed out, much of this damage could be eliminated by seat belts properly worn.

It is difficult to avoid accidents with the majority of children's activities by such measures as wearing mouth protectors. When they are worn in such sports as rugby football, soccer (perhaps), boxing and other short duration games, the effects are very good. But one can hardly say to a child, 'You are going out to play Cops and Robbers with your friends are you? Well, you'd better put in this mouth shield.'

It would be foolish for a child to wear anything like that while swimming. The number of dental accidents in swimming pools is unbelievable and it is difficult to understand how they happen. Youngsters will tell you that they hit the bottom in a dive before they knew it, but it is difficult to see how the top front teeth are damaged in this way. Much more acceptable is the explanation that in emerging from the pool the wet hands slipped on the side and the mouth crashed down on the edge of the pool or the hand rail. The best way to avoid such accidents, as with others, is to warn children that they can happen and to be careful. But it is natural for children to play and forget the rules and so we must be prepared for accidents. Perhaps it is a move in the right direction, although some sports lovers object, that protective helmets are being worn by cricketers. If they work it will help to reduce some of the more frightening casualties caused by the bullet-like ball striking the brave but foolhardy batsman in the face. Mouth protectors should be worn in the following contact sports: hockey, soccer, rugby, boxing, squash, lacrosse, and basketball. Ask your dentist for the details of suitable models for any of these pursuits. Prevention is best.

What to do when accidents happen

First of all, remember not to panic. If the accident happens to a child, especially your child, there will be a tendency to feel helpless and scared, but this will convey itself to the victim and it will be difficult then to carry out any sensible first aid treatment. Although the first thing that may be apparent is a bleeding mouth and broken tooth or teeth, it is essential to find out whether there is any other injury which may need more urgent treatment than the broken teeth. Thus a quick examination is necessary and after that you should deal with the bleeding. Make sure that the blood is not being swallowed or inhaled. In the case of the unconscious victim the mouth should be cleared of blood, the head turned on one side and the tongue pulled forward to make sure that the victim can breathe.

We do not propose here to go into all the aspects of first aid because this will be found in any simple first aid book and copies *should* be readily available in every home. So, Rule No. 1, if a child presents with a condition where a tooth has been knocked out, it is important to try and find that tooth. Carefully rinse it – don't scrub – and place it in something wet, plain water will do, or the child's saliva; milk is better still. The tooth should be kept moist until dental advice can be obtained, which should be as soon as possible. Where there are cracked teeth with portions left in the gum, try to find all the pieces in order to make sure there are no remaining fragments of teeth, embedded in the lip perhaps.

If the teeth are displaced, either pushed forward or pushed back towards the back of the palate, it is important to try and very quickly realign them and hold them there for a few seconds with a clean handkerchief, a piece of gauze or other clean cloth. In all these cases the quicker one gets dental advice, the better. Where teeth have broken off, and after blood has gently been wiped from around the teeth (be careful, the teeth may be very sensitive), try to see whether there is any evidence of dental pulp showing inside the broken edge of tooth. That is, has the fracture gone across the pulp? This can be seen by a red area in the middle of the tooth which itself may be bleeding. In such a case URGENT treatment will be necessary, first of all to relieve the victim of pain and also to try and save the tooth. Remember that teeth which have been knocked out can be reinserted, and experience has shown that it is important to get the tooth back into its socket within thirty minutes of the accident. The chances of the tooth 'taking' and being retained are very high. Usually the life of such teeth is up to five years, but much longer if replaced immediately. This may be valuable time gained, during which the jaw grows and space is kept while other treatment can be planned.

The following rules are suggested:

1. Calm yourself.

2. Calm the victim, whether child or adult.

3. Gently cover any fractured tooth with a small piece of clean moist cotton wool or gauze, preferably soaked in a weak salt solution.

4. Preserve any tooth which has been knocked out in saliva, wetted gauze or fresh milk and keep it moist until you see the dentist. Preferably replace immediately back in its socket.

5. Get in touch with a dentist and explain the urgency of the problem. If you cannot be seen immediately, it is worth a journey to the nearest hospital where the casualty department is geared for such an eventuality. Make sure there are dental staff available because expert advice and attention are needed. The *medical* casualty officer may not feel strongly about saving a tooth and if the child is otherwise reasonably fit, the dental problem may not be

attended to. The dental surgeon will probably wish to take radiographs around the area to see that the supporting bone has not been damaged and also that portions of tooth have not been left in the lip.

There will almost certainly be swelling for a day or so, but this will clear up and any cuts, unless they are very wide, will heal up. On the other hand, a deep cut may need stitching and this should be done by the dentist or at the dental hospital. If the tooth (and it is usually a front tooth) has been fractured at the biting edge and the pulp does not seem to be directly involved, you may safely wait a day before the dentist sees it. In nearly all these cases the dentist will make a cover of some sort to protect the damaged portion of the tooth, and if the damage is unsightly, he will eventually construct a restoration which will reproduce the shape of the original tooth. However, do not expect a perfect crown to be permanently fixed until the child is eighteen and almost full growth has occurred.

In the aftercare one needs patience but in the immediate instance a considerable amount of help can be given. Everything should settle down within a few days. If the damage is very severe the dentist may have to remove the pulp but this is done quite painlessly under a local anaesthetic or, if the child is very anxious, it may be done while the child has a general anaesthetic for a few minutes while the pulp is removed and the tooth has a root filling, and eventually a crown can be fitted.

More serious accidents such as *fracture of the jaw* require specialized hospital treatment, but in the meantime the important point to remember is again, no panic. Next, try to immobilize the jaws – that is, keep them fixed in the closed position if possible. Often it is difficult to close the jaws, but keep them as closed as possible and one of the things that can help is to wind a bandage round the top of the head and jaw fairly gently, but firmly, so that the jaws are held together, but make sure that no blood is at the back of the throat. This is always the most important point in any accident. A fractured jaw is an emergency and requires very quick attention because the earlier the condition is treated the easier the jaw can be set in the correct position and the quicker healing occurs.

Sometimes people *dislocate* their jaws with a wide yawn or

perhaps trying to chew a large portion of food. With some people the jaw dislocates very easily. The jaws no longer come together in the usual manner, but seem to be propped up at the back of the mouth with the teeth widely separated. It is possible to reduce these dislocations very easily, but care has to be taken by the person who is doing it, because the lower jaw can snap back into position very quickly and your fingers could be severely bitten.

What you do is to wrap some towelling around both index fingers, place both thumbs under the back of each jaw and the two index fingers on top of the bottom back teeth and by pressing the index fingers downwards and the thumbs upwards the jaw will then go into place but this *must* be done with care. When the jaw has gone back into place it will be obvious that things are corrected. There will be some soreness perhaps for a couple of hours, but this will disappear. It is advisable for those who experience frequent dislocation of their jaws to take advice from a dentist who may refer the patient to a specialist.

Bleeding

Bleeding tooth sockets may occur at home at any time following extraction, very occasionally when the local anaesthetic has worn off. If you have a tendency to bleed, or one of your family has a tendency to bleed, your dentist must be told about it if ever he contemplates removing a tooth.

He will then take precautions and may administer certain medicaments which will prevent or minimize the bleeding. If there is a history of haemophilia or other bleeding in the family the dentist *must* be told and will refer the patient to a clinic which is organized for the special precautions which can be taken for such patients.

Bleeding from the mouth after extraction requires the following attention:

1. Again no panic.
2. The more you rinse the more you will bleed. So the minimum of rinsing.
3. If the mouth is full of clot, this should be wiped free very gently and the area from which the bleeding is coming should be noted and a large piece of gauze, three-inch square, or a clean handkerchief should be folded up and placed over the bleeding

area and the patient instructed to bite down hard on this for about fifteen minutes with as much pressure as possible. At the end of this time the area can be examined. Usually the bleeding has stopped or has diminished considerably. Some people panic when they spit out and see a pink/red fluid. This is blood-stained saliva, and is of no consequence. If after fifteen minutes the bleeding has not stopped by pressure on the gauze, one might try using a teabag which has been moistened and wrung out and placed with the gauze and bitten on. The small amount of tannic acid in tea should help to control the bleeding but, remember, NO RINSING if you can help it. Any clots can be wiped away and gauze applied. You should never try to pack any gauze or cotton into the socket. If bleeding does not stop, the dentist should be contacted as soon as possible, but in most cases pressure will control bleeding. This happens in most parts of the body and there is no reason why it should not happen in the mouth. However, there are some points which one should remember. Aspirin tends to promote bleeding so it is wise to use other pain relief if it's needed. Pressure to stop bleeding must be applied at the point of bleeding: squeezing the edges of the socket together is of great value.

It would be wise to list in your telephone notebook any local hospital which maintains a round-the-clock dental service. This is very rare, even in big cities. There are now some area emergency dental services run by teams of dentists and it is worth making a note of their telephone numbers but remember that these emergency services may be costly if used outside working hours.

Facial injury and motor accidents

The use of seat belts will substantially reduce the severity of facial injury resulting from accident. The injuries are usually caused by impact with the panel or windscreen. But injuries resulting from crashes are dealt with by the appropriate hospital units (facial injuries are usually treated by maxillo-facial teams) and are therefore beyond the scope of this book.

Self-imposed damage

Teeth can be damaged by using them as instruments or tools so do *not* use them to:

1. Open kirby grips (bobby pins).
2. Remove bottle caps.
3. Bite through thread.
4. Crack nuts.
5. Manicure – nail biting has been shown to damage lower front teeth!

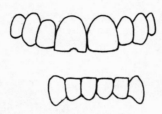

Figure 14. Upper front teeth are often chipped in this way by biting cotton or opening hair grips.

10
The Good Dentist

'How do I find a good dentist?'

This is a question that is always being asked and it crops up frequently when dentistry is discussed in radio 'phone-in' programmes. It is impossible to give a reasonable answer. It would be simple to answer the question 'How do I find a dentist?' But finding a *good* dentist is as difficult as finding a *good* lawyer, or doctor, or a *good* electrician, motor mechanic, TV repair man, plumber. The problem is the definition of 'good'. What does anyone mean by it? I suppose on the whole it means the person who gives honest, prompt service at reasonable cost. That would be fair for most of the services mentioned above, but with dentistry there are a number of other considerations because of the close personal contact between the parties. Only with a dentist could the 'customer' be put off by personal considerations such as smelly breath or tobacco-stained fingers. It doesn't matter if the plumber has a rude, unpleasant manner so long as the burst pipes are repaired expeditiously.

What advice should I give the members of the public? Again I must hedge and be vague. So many factors are involved. We all have good and bad days and you and the dentist may meet on a day when he has been overwhelmed by emergencies and no matter how much he tries he may be unable to give you the attention that you need and deserve. The considerate patient may note the probable unusual circumstances of *that* day and decide to give the dentist another chance, but another person may decide to go elsewhere, telling friends, 'Don't go there, the place is chaotic.'

Here are a few tips for finding a *good* dentist.

1. *Ask some friends* whose judgement you think you can trust. Each will give a name and probably some of these friends will be enthusiastic. Remember, however, to ask what that dentist *does*. If you require a full set of false teeth and your friend is ecstatic about his jacket crown work you may be on to the wrong man. If your friend's dentist is described as doing everything well, make sure when you telephone for an appointment that you give a short description of the sort of attention you require – a general check-up, new false teeth, children's dentistry, orthodontics (straightening teeth), preventive dentistry. It may save you from an embarrassing and fruitless visit. After all, doctors differ in their specialities and interests and you would not dream of going to see a gynaecologist about your flat feet.

Even very intelligent people are not able to judge the level of the treatment they have been receiving. Patients may say to their new dentist, 'I've come to you because my own marvellous dentist, who has been looking after me for twenty years, has now retired. He really was a wonderful chap and I hope you will be able to do as well as he has done.' Examination often reveals a mouth in an appalling state of breakdown although the patient has attended regularly twice a year. We call this 'supervised neglect'. The patient has been pleased with the 'treatment' because it has always been quick and painless. Any pain which has occurred between visits (due to this neglect) has often been dealt with by the simple expedient of extracting the offending tooth.

On the other hand, the opposite situation may occur in which a patient may attend complaining bitterly about the 'expensive' dentist who 'takes ages' over his work. Dentists often find here that excellent care of a very high standard has been performed and they may try hard to persuade the patient to return to the previous dentist. However, that is not always possible because of other considerations such as personality clashes.

The sad fact is that very often the quality of dentistry is a minor consideration where friends are recommending. The main criterion is 'he does not hurt, ever'.

2. *Ask your doctor.* This would seem to be the most sensible way of finding a good dentist. But many have had very poor treatment themselves, mainly because they have taken too little care of their mouths and because their work has caused their attendance to be

irregular. They have not been very cooperative patients. The lack of knowledge of the mouth on the part of many doctors is unbelievable, but on the other hand many are capable of giving good advice because they might have heard 'good and bad opinions' from other medical men and dentists which will enable them to make a judgement. So it is worth asking your family doctor for a recommendation. One of the advantages of such a recommendation is that the very busy dentist, who may not otherwise be able to fit you in, will try hard to please a professional colleague if you mention that Dr Whatsisname recommended you to call.

3. *Ask a dentist.* We are back where we began. I mentioned to you that this is a question frequently asked by strangers. The truth is that we know of good dentists, but would be very hazy about the capabilities of a dentist in another part of the country. I have even been asked by a patient to give him the name of a good dentist in a small town in South Carolina! (The answer is to *go there* and go through the same procedure as we are now describing for home-based patients.)

You cannot ask your previous dentist if you have left him after some disagreement, but if you have moved to another district he *may* know of a colleague who has a good reputation for the sort of work you require.

4. *Ask at a dental teaching hospital.* If there is one that is near where you live, or intend living, and you need some special attention (such as gum/periodontal treatment) you might be able to telephone the relevant department at that dental hospital and ask a member of staff whether he knows of a dentist in the area who could deal with the problem. It may be better to write in with your query once you have found out by your telephone call the correct person to whom to address your letter.

If you have children it is essential that the dentist you approach (a) is willing to treat children and (b) believes in preventive dentistry above all else. Make sure about this when you telephone for an appointment for your children. You will not necessarily find a good dentist by counting the letters after his name, although extra qualifications may be important if you require specialist treatment. You won't be helped, either, by sticking a pin in the yellow pages or even the Dentists' Register. A dentist who has a part-time hospital appointment may be very good, or he may be a good teacher and has taken a hospital appointment to fill in his vacant practice time. The addition of the title 'Dr' in front of a dentist's name does not necessarily make him any better either!

From the above you can see there is no certain way of finding a good dentist. It may be difficult enough to get an appointment with *any* dentist and you can be sure that good dentists (like good theatre shows or restaurants) will be in great demand. You have to be prepared to try the dentist who seems, from all you have heard, to suit you best. Then it all depends on how you get on together.

Terms used to describe dental specialists

Endodontist	One who specializes in the treatment of the root canals of teeth.
Oral surgeon	One who undertakes surgical procedures of the mouth and jaws.
Orthodontist	One who treats irregularities of the teeth and jaw relationship.
Paedodontist	One who treats the teeth and mouths of children.
Periodontist	One who treats the gums and other supporting tissues of the teeth.
Prosthodontist	One who plans and fits replacement teeth.

Check on your dentist

Do any of the following apply to your dentist?

1. Doesn't take regular radiographs. Even when he does, he doesn't consult them when working.

2. No medical/dental history taken. Makes no note of the pills/medicines you are taking.

3. Surgery not clean.

4. No assistants.

5. No topical anaesthetic applied before local anaesthetic. Doesn't wait for injection to work.

6. Doesn't explain things to you.

7. No treatment plan to discuss.

8. Doesn't see you in emergency time.

9. Always late. Dismisses you on the stroke of time whether your job is completed or not.

10. Talks about fees rather than work.

11. Suggests a lot of fillings when you have been passed okay by someone else.

12. Tells you there is nothing wrong when you have been told there is lots to do.

13. Tells you your pain is 'imagined' after a cursory examination.

14. Doesn't mention prevention, just fills holes as they appear.

15. Does a five-minute scale and clean/brush around. Never takes more than one visit to clean your teeth.

16. Doesn't gently probe your gums for periodontal pockets at your check-up.

17. No disposables.

18. Boils his instruments (an inefficient method of sterilizing).

19. Does root canal treatments without use of rubber dam.

We are treading on dangerous ground here. Dental treatment is a matter of personal choice of premises and design. The smartest and most elegant surgeries do not guarantee good standards. They could be a front for poor treatment. One or two omissions above may be of no consequence, but if too many are noticeable, you probably have grounds for some concern.

11
Attending the Dentist

Making the appointment

When you telephone for an appointment it is important to give the secretary the following information:

New Patient: Full name, address, telephone number where you can be reached during the day (this is essential in case the dentist is ill or called away), the name of the person who recommended you and the reason for your appointment. It may be for a routine examination to check that everything is fine, or you may have an urgent problem – toothache or an unsightly broken front tooth. Tell the secretary if you are in pain and she will make sure you are given an appointment without delay. Remember that you may be 'squeezed' into an already full book and therefore not only will a rapid appointment mean that you might be kept a while in the waiting-room, but that the following patient may also be delayed by your problem.

State the purpose of your visit as clearly as you can. It could be that the dentist who has been recommended to you does not carry out the sort of treatment you want. For example, you require a complete set of artificial teeth and the dentist does not make dentures. If this is explained the secretary may recommend another dentist who does.

Dentistry, like medicine, has become more and more complex so that many dentists limit their work to that part which they do best. Be sure before you make the appointment that you have the right man! In many countries the dentist has a choice whether he operates under a subsidized service, e.g. Medicare, Medicaid or the National Health Service, or privately. MAKE IT CLEAR BEFORE YOU GET YOUR APPOINTMENT if you want treatment under such a subsidized scheme, if available, otherwise you may find yourself attending a private practice.

Routine revisit 'old' patient: As above, state your full name, address – give the old address as well as any new address and telephone number if you have moved since your last series of visits. Say whether you are coming for a regular examination or for specific treatment and if possible give the time since your last visit. If there is more than one dentist in the practice, or you see a hygienist on your routine visits, state the name of the person who attended to you last. All this will help the practice to get all your records ready in time for your visit.

If you have been referred by another dentist it may be useful to bring along any X-ray films that you have or ask the referring dentist to send any that may be helpful. The X-ray films themselves do not belong to the patient, but to the dentist who took them. He charged you for the service and the diagnosis and report on them, not for the actual plates (see page 72 on X-rays).

Missing your appointment. If you are in business and you miss a day at work your produce can always be sold another day. But the dentist has only his skill and his *time* with which to earn his living. Once 'lost' the time can never be made up again. It costs a great deal to maintain a practice – bearing in mind staff salaries, rent and other overhead expenses. Therefore, if you cannot keep an appointment you *must* give fair warning so that the time can be filled in. The dentist usually asks for twenty-four hours, but three to four hours is better than nothing. Even if he cannot fill in the time with patients he can, if he knows you can't come, occupy himself with other important tasks. But if he has to sit down doing nothing while waiting for you, knowing that other patients have telephoned for urgent attention, he is likely to be rather put out! Also he is entitled to charge a fair fee for his lost time.

If you think you might be a few minutes late, telephone and explain the delay and check whether it will still be reasonable to keep the appointment. If the dentist is very occupied it may suit you both to make another date, so be reasonable and understanding. It will pay dividends in good relationship for you both.

In our own practice we separate the 'good' from the 'bad'. The habitual appointment-breakers eventually find it difficult to get an appointment at all. Remember, a dentist's lost time is like today's newspaper. It cannot be sold tomorrow.

Arriving on time. It is important to keep to the time you were given. Some patients say, 'Well, the dentist keeps me waiting sometimes, so I can't see why I shouldn't keep him waiting. I'm in business and when he keeps me waiting I lose time, too.'

There is a difference. The dentist is a member of a healing profession and may be dealing with people in pain and distress. His carefully-made appointment schedule may be disrupted by all kinds of untoward events – a little boy hit in the face by a swing, an unexpected difficulty with an emergency extraction, another patient coming late because of a delayed train. The dentist who never keeps you waiting may be a remarkably organized person. It may also be that he never sees emergencies or it may be that he sends away patients who come a few minutes late even if they have travelled fifty miles. Would you like that to happen to you? It is impossible to be completely accurate about how long any dental procedure will take. Sometimes what looks like a simple filling turns out to be more involved and if the patient has had an injected local anaesthetic to numb the tooth it is better to go on and finish the job if possible.

The most cooperative patients get the best work done. If the dentist is harassed he cannot work at his best.

If you are a new patient and you are desperately anxious or nervous, tell the receptionist or nurse and you will discover that modern dentistry has many ways of making your visit smooth and free from stress. But remember that no dentist is going to work on you the moment you step into his room. He must examine you carefully and make a plan of any treatment required and he will discuss this with you. Later, if you are having pain, he will attend to that after finding out the cause.

What to say to the dentist

It is important to give the dentist a history of your trouble. What is the main reason for coming? Usually the good dentist will ask you all the relevant questions to ensure that everything he will do or use will be suitable for your condition.

If I myself were to walk into a dental practice and the dentist wanted to do something to my teeth without finding out my dental/medical history I would not be satisfied. Many of us today are on special medicaments for chronic conditions – the dentist *must* know about them before he does anything!

So, tell him about yourself. He should know the following:

Have you had any serious illnesses?
What were they?
Are you fit now?
Have you ever had a general anaesthetic?
What for?
Are you a bleeder?
Have you ever bled excessively after an extraction?
Or had any nosebleeds?
Have you ever had rheumatic fever even years ago as a child?
Are you on any regular medicines?
Anti-coagulants?
Gout pills, pills for high blood pressure?
How *is* your blood pressure?
Are you on the birth control pill?
Is there any diabetes in your immediate family?
Are you allergic to anything?
Or do you have hay fever or asthma?
Did penicillin give you a rash?
Do you smoke?

Some people have pacemakers to regulate the heart beat and are otherwise fit. This must be mentioned to the dentist as some electrical apparatus may upset the action of the pacemaker.

These are just some of the facts any dentist should know. In the light of some of your answers he may modify the type of work he does and the way he does it.

For example, it is accepted that if you have had rheumatic fever you should have scaling or extractions carried out under antibiotic cover. The dentist will arrange for you to have antibiotics just before starting such a procedure.

If you have high blood pressure and are on tablets like Propanalol (Inderal) he may use a different kind of injection.

Do not get upset if the dentist asks you a lot of questions and think, 'Why doesn't he get on with the dentistry?' He is caring for you as a person – your health and safety are more important than the restoration of a tooth.

Dos and don'ts for your first visit

1. Even if you are very nervous do not drink alcohol before you attend. When he smells the booze the dentist may easily mark your chart 'alcoholic – special care'. Of course, if you *are* an alcoholic it doesn't matter much – your teeth won't last too long anyway!

2. Stay away from the onions and garlic the day before.

3. Some dentists allow smoking in their waiting-rooms, which they consider the private untouchable preserve of the patient; other dentists do not. If other patients in the waiting-room object, it is courteous to give in. However, never try to smoke when entering the consulting room. You will be pushed out very quietly.

4. Do brush your teeth *gently* and carefully before attending even if you have never brushed before.

Some patients feel guilty about this and brush like mad just before they come in and all we see is a mass of torn, inflamed gums. Don't worry, be gentle and the dentist or hygienist will show you how to brush your teeth effectively and tenderly. It helps to take along your usual toothbrush on your first visit. It can then be checked to see whether it is suitable and how you use it. Do not, whatever you do, buy a new toothbrush before your visit. It may not be what the dentist thinks is correct for you.

Don't be suspicious or show lack of confidence. Confidence breeds confidence.

Don't worry. It will be all right. Much, much better than you thought.

Don't funk it at the last moment. You are cheating yourself and the dentist.

12
Avoiding Pain

Probably fewer than fifty per cent of the eligible population attend for regular dental care. The remainder wait until they are driven by desperation to have emergency treatment such as extractions. Dentistry in the modern age is unlikely to be painful and almost all procedures can be carried out with little discomfort; yet the fear of pain is still the main cause of dental neglect. Pain itself is a mystery and not well understood, but its elimination during operations has successfully been accomplished. The extent of pain is influenced by a number of factors and it is well known that there are different levels of pain tolerance for different people. Some can calmly put up with a level of pain which would have others screaming for relief. This assumes that both are feeling the same amount of pain, and pain can be measured by certain scientific methods.

On the other hand, the level of pain differs not only among people, as any dentist knows, but also among the teeth themselves. Thus, in the pre-anaesthetic days there were many patients who did not feel the tooth being drilled and even today there are those who will refuse a local anaesthetic for a filling because they say it doesn't bother them. Of course some of these refusals are because the patient fears the needle more than the drill!

Try a little experiment. Tweak the skin on the back of your left hand between the finger nails of the thumb and middle finger of your right hand. You did it without flinching: The entry of the needle is less than this, so why are so many of us worried about the injection? The first answer is probably a built-in biological resistance to the entry of foreign objects into one's body.

I remember as a child of about five needing to have a series of weekly injections. I can still recall the tremendous resistance I put up to the first one and how, after that, I hardly noticed my regular dose. I must have been particularly fortunate because the second reason for the fear of injections is the genuinely remembered pain inflicted by injections of olden days – the blunt needle, the clumsy operator and possibly the post-injection infection. The introduction of the 'use once' disposable needle ensures sharpness and safety from sepsis. The clumsy operator probably exists in all areas of work, but is fortunately fairly rare in the qualified dentists of today.

Most of the work dentists do for you does not need anaesthetics of any sort, especially if you attend regularly for a check-up. With modern preventive methods there will be little to be done except possibly scaling and cleaning. So the moral is, the more confidence you have the less there will be to fear. Conversely, the longer fear makes you neglect regular care, the more treatment will eventually be necessary, with the need for anaesthetics.

Assuming your dentist is going to carry out some procedure which might be uncomfortable, what methods can be used for pain prevention? The choice can be from the following:

1. Local anaesthesia (injection): patient stays awake.

2. General anaesthesia: patient goes to sleep. Either intravenous (IV) injection usually into the arm or inhalation (gas).

3. Relative analgesia. Inhalation of nitrous oxide (gas) which acts as a sedative. Patient does not go to sleep. Local anaesthetic may be used as well.

4. Hypnosis.

1. *Local anaesthesia.* The gum area around the tooth is injected with Lignocaine through a fine needle and there is complete numbness after a few minutes.

Another form of local anaesthesia is block anaesthesia where the nerve to one quadrant of the jaw (usually the lower jaw) is 'deadened' by injection at the back of the jaw. This may be necessary in the lower jaw because the bone is very dense and the solution deposited under the gum around the tooth may not soak through the bone to the nerves of the tooth. The injection at the back of the jaw reaches the nerve before it enters the bone.

What makes injections so much more comfortable today? There is the use of fine disposable needles and the application of numbing liquids or pastes on the gum prior to injection. These are called *topical* or *surface* anaesthetics and are very important for making injections almost imperceptible. If you are going to have an injection in the mouth ask for a 'topical' first. This is painted on the gum above the tooth and left to take effect for about two minutes – the time lag is important. After this the entry of the needle should be unnoticed.

The dentist makes the injection more comfortable by injecting *slowly* because quick injection stretches the tissues. The dentist may inject one drop into the tissue very quickly and wait for this to work (he may remove the syringe and reinsert it a minute or two later into a quite painless area). Sometimes patients ask for 'lots of injection to make sure the tooth is quite numb'. The judgement of the dentist should be relied on here. If you have more injection than is really necessary the numb feeling will take longer to wear off, which can be a nuisance if you are going out for a meal, and a great deal of anaesthetic is more likely to be a cause of after-pain when the numbness wears off. Usually when the teeth are anaesthetized the lip on the same side goes numb and sometimes, for lower teeth, the tongue too. For the duration of the numbness you must be careful about eating (preferably do not eat), as you might bite your tongue or lips without knowing it. It may take one hour or more with a block anaesthetic for the effects to wear off.

Don't forget to tell the dentist if you have any unusual medical history or are taking any tablets or medicines, e.g. anti-depressant drugs. He may vary the make-up of the type of local anaesthetic he injects.

Do not expect topical anaesthetics from your doctor before injections under the skin. They do not work on the skin.

2. *General anaesthesia.* Local anaesthetics are generally very sure and are the safest and best way for the dentist to work. Just occasionally a local anaesthetic may not work satisfactorily because something is preventing the drug from penetrating to the nerve. This is usually associated with severe inflammation around the tooth or perhaps an abscess where there is throbbing and swelling. In the latter event the dentist would not want to inject into the infected area around the tooth in case he spreads the infection. In these circumstances he may recommend general anaesthesia by intravenous injection into the arm or by inhalation anaesthetic (gas) breathed in through a mask over the nose. If you are going to

sleep, the dentist should not act as both operator (i.e. working on your tooth) and anaesthetist. Don't allow it in any circumstances! I would not allow it for myself or members of my family and would not expect others to be so treated. In cases of abscesses requiring urgent attention it may be possible to delay the operation until the infection has subsided by the use of antibiotics. However, if the dentist can use the services of another dentist or doctor, so much the better. Of course, the ideal is where the anaesthetic is administered under the care of a specialist anaesthetist, but this is not always necessary and in practice may cause delay and extra expense.

For general anaesthetics the following precautions must be observed. This applies to all cases where you go to sleep for however short a time.

i. Your general physical condition must be known to the dentist and anaesthetist.

ii. NOTHING, repeat NOTHING, must be taken by mouth for a full *four hours* before the anaesthetic is given. This means no food or drink – not even water or aspirin. Otherwise the effect of the anaesthetic may cause vomiting and that would be most undesirable.

iii. Remember to empty the bladder and bowels before the operation.

iv. Never drive to the appointment unless you have someone with you to drive the car home. You must NOT DRIVE again that day after a general (not local) anaesthetic, or use complicated machinery.

v. Always have someone meet and accompany you home no matter how well you feel.

For a general anaesthetic of long duration, such as may be required for removal of wisdom teeth, it is better for the dentist to arrange for you to go to a hospital with after-care facilities. In these circumstances it is usually the plan to have, say, all the wisdom teeth removed if necessary at the one operation.

Anaesthetics (usually Brietal – in the USA Brevital) may be injected into the arm or other conveniently accessible vein. In less than a minute the patient becomes pleasantly unconscious and the operation proceeds after packs are placed in the back of the mouth to make sure that nothing slips down the throat while the patient is unconscious. For longer anaesthetics a tube may be passed down the throat into the windpipe (while the patient is asleep) for greater safety. This usually occurs when the patient is having the anaesthetic in hospital. On regaining consciousness the throat may be sore occasionally.

Some operations, not necessarily serious, such as the preparation of front teeth for crowns, or operations on the gums all round the mouth may be so prolonged that some patients could become anxious, although most do not worry as long as they feel no pain. For added comfort the long procedure may be carried out under intravenous Valium (diazepam). This is injected into a vein in the arm; the patient does not become unconscious, but feels very pleasantly relaxed. The area to be operated on has a local anaesthetic injection for numbness and however long the operation takes, the patient has very little awareness of time elapsed.

Intravenous Valium is very much appreciated by patients and since there is no unconsciousness it is safer than general anaesthetics. Because of the deep relaxation many of the precautions regarding health checks should be observed; the four-hour fasting before administration is not essential but there should be abstention from food and drink for an hour or two.

3. *Relative analgesia.* This is a method of relaxation very popular in the USA. It is the administration by nasal mask of nitrous oxide (gas) with high oxygen mixture. The patient has this continuously while drilling, etc., is being done and most are completely relaxed. Local injections are used around the teeth at the same time. The drawback here is that special equipment is needed to ensure that the required dosage of gas is not exceeded. Also, not all patients respond in the same way and in fact there seems to be a psychological element involved. However, most of the patients who have experienced this method of relaxation ask for it again. Precautions regarding eating and drinking should be observed for two hours before relative analgesia.

Dentists who have been using this technique routinely have been warned in the USA that the level of gas in their operating rooms may accumulate and can have a harmful effect upon the staff if it continues over long periods of time. Thus, there is some concern that all practices in which this technique is used frequently should have some method of air conditioning or air exchange. The *patient* of course is not at risk.

4. *Hypnosis.* Many dentists have attended courses on medical hypnosis, but in the main it is not extensively used in general practice. Hypnosis is kept in reserve as just another technique which might be used for the patient's comfort. However, the effect on the dentist who has practised hypnosis is that eventually his whole manner is one of suggestion which relaxes the nervous patient. The disadvantage of hypnosis is that one is never sure who will make a good subject. Those who are amenable to suggestion under hypnosis have had teeth out and fillings made without anaesthetics.

There is no doubt that in spite of all the sedations and anaesthetics, some of which have been mentioned above, the dentist will do his best work and the patient will fare best and be safest when work is done under local anaesthesia, i.e. numbing only the tooth or teeth. Make this the first choice if you can and if the dentist agrees. If you are very nervous tell your dentist and he will see that you are made comfortable and relaxed before he does anything. A tablet or two of a premedication drug (this may be a tranquillizer) about half an hour before the work commences may be all you need to give you confidence. When it comes to a discussion about having a general anaesthetic many factors have to be considered, especially that of economics. If the dentist decides that a certain treatment is best carried out at hospital the cost of the bed is important as well.

13
The Mother and Child

Pregnancy

There are vast numbers of old wives' tales about pregnancy and teeth. And so, without any further ado, let us assert that pregnancy does NOT cause your teeth to go bad. This contradicts the tale that every pregnancy means the loss of a tooth. After the doctor has confirmed the happy event-to-be, the expectant mother (who often has a job as well as housework to do) is involved in a multitude of extra activities such as attending the ante-natal clinic, buying baby clothes, perhaps altering the home to accommodate baby. It is therefore understandable that she may put off seeing the dentist about her teeth. With the arrival of baby she is more tied than before and it may be a year or two before the dentist is seen. Besides neglecting her own dental care she may succumb to the lure of sweets and other carbohydrate foods. In time, therefore, there may well be dental troubles, but they are not due to the pregnancy. Two conditions can arise: dental decay, which can commonly occur in pregnancy around the parts of the teeth level with the gum, and gingivitis where the gums themselves become red and swollen and bleed easily. Neither of these need arise if the following precautions are taken:

1. The dentist (and he may refer the expectant mother to his hygienist for instruction in maintaining mouth health for herself and the baby) should be visited as early as possible in the first stages of pregnancy for a thorough examination so that all necessary treatment can be carried out well in advance. This is important, for later on the dentist may not have time to complete any necessary fillings and may have to put in temporary dressings.

This may lead to problems later in pregnancy or even during confinement. The best and safest time for any extensive treatment is during the middle three months.

2. The doctor should advise a suitable diet pattern to protect the mother-to-be and also the developing child. The dentist, or especially the dental hygienist if there is one available, will also discuss diet in relation to preserving the health of the teeth and gums and also to help develop sound teeth in the baby. In that respect the doctor should avoid, if at all possible, the prescribing of tetracycline antibiotics for expectant mothers and for infants, as they are likely to cause serious discolouration of the child's teeth.

Essentially the mother's diet should include all the proteins, minerals and vitamins which the foetus needs. In order to meet the added needs of calcium and phosphorus for bone and tooth development, sufficient milk or milk products per day should be consumed. A recommended list would look something like this:

> *Proteins*: meat, eggs, fish and poultry.
> *Vegetables*: greens, cabbage, sprouts, etc., for Vitamin A and iron.
> *Citrus fruits*: oranges, lemons, grapefruit.

It is important to reduce the amount of foods which contain sugars (sucrose) so as to control excess weight and to prevent dental decay.

The developing child does not remove calcium from the mother's teeth. Any breakdown of the teeth is due to the usual causes, perhaps accentuated by the conditions above. But minerals such as calcium and phosphorus can be removed from the mother's bones and the bone around the teeth. Thus the diet must contain sufficient of these minerals to prevent loss from the bones. There is still very little confirmed evidence that the addition of fluoride to the mother's diet influences the formation of the teeth in the foetus.

Bleeding and Swollen Gums can be common during pregnancy. There are hormonal changes during this time, so that any neglect of the mouth leaving bacteria around the teeth might cause a mild inflammation which tends to be worse during pregnancy. However, if attention is paid to thorough cleansing of the teeth there is no likelihood of 'pregnancy gingivitis' occurring. There may be some improvement in the gum condition after the birth of the child, but remember that the trouble was there before pregnancy and will not clear up completely until expert advice has been obtained. Sometimes a single enlargement of the gum occurs, perhaps related to one or two teeth. The lump bleeds easily and may interfere with eating. It has been called a pregnancy 'tumour'. A similar condition may occur with those on the contraceptive pill, the effect of which is to mimic the pregnant state.

It is not really a tumour so there is no need to be seriously worried about it. The dentist can deal with it quite easily. He may decide, however, to delay treatment until after the birth of the baby. But, it should be stressed again, it does not have to occur and will not in the scrupulously looked after mouth.

When people have bleeding gums they often allow the condition to worsen because they deliberately keep the toothbrush away from the part of the mouth where the gums bleed. Thus, because there is an accumulation of plaque the bleeding will get worse. If you take your soft brush firmly in your hand and brush away, especially in the area that bleeds, the gums will improve after a day or so. If you are afraid to do this try taking a clean piece of cloth (a thin, clean piece of towelling wrapped around the finger will be fine) and rub this over the teeth and gums. The use of disclosing solutions, or tablets (ask your chemist), will show whether you have successfully removed enough of the layers of germ colonies to do the trick (every day).

The new baby

At birth there are no teeth showing in the mouth, but the first teeth are forming under the gums. The saliva glands are not formed until about six months and when the baby starts to salivate more it does not necessarily mean that the baby's teeth are starting to erupt. However, the appearance of the first baby tooth at around five and a half to six months does usually coincide with the onset of salivation and dribbling! That is why it is inadvisable to give your baby regular solids as a diet until this time. Not because he or she cannot chew them without teeth, but because there may not be enough saliva to moisten them and enable them to be swallowed comfortably. Just try eating a dry biscuit without a drink afterwards to wash it down. Occasionally babies are born with one or two teeth in place, usually the lower front ones. This is not a sign from God nor does it indicate that the baby is exceptionally advanced. The teeth have relatively little root formation and are fortunately lost after a few days. (They could make breast feeding uncomfortable!)

The average ages for the eruption of primary, milk or baby teeth are given on p. 17. 'Teething' may give some discomfort as the teeth break through the gums. You can see the bumps in the gums which may appear red. Also the child's cheeks may be red and hot. Usually a spoonful of paracetamol (acetominophen) paediatric elixir will do the trick if the baby is very hot and uncomfortable and sometimes (rarely) the family doctor could be called in. But baby soon gets over it until the next tooth comes through. It's usually all over by the age of two.

The mother should not compare the time of eruption or shedding of her children's teeth with those of neighbours or friends. There is a wide variation, and early or late eruption generally means very little. If a friend's child has a first tooth at five months and yours does not show signs of anything until eight months it does not mean that the other baby is more advanced. It is just part of life's variation. It is important not to fret about things like that. One of the prime causes of worry is when mothers phone and say, 'My child's second tooth is growing up behind the first one which is still there.' This often happens and is no cause for worry. The first tooth will soon be shed and the position of the second tooth *behind it* is normal in most cases.

Feeding your child

Breast-feeding

Doctors prefer the mother to breast-feed the new baby. There are many reasons for this, the most important being that the baby thus shares some of the immunity acquired by the mother against various diseases. Immunity factors are passed into the milk and so the baby has an added resistance for the first weeks of life.

From the dental viewpoint all the necessary balanced nutrients are in the mother's milk so that the jaws and teeth can develop satisfactorily. The act of sucking is moreover of great importance to proper development. There is strong action of the tongue and pressure on the jaws and lips and these are then stimulated by the effort the child makes to obtain milk. Unfortunately most bottles for babies do not give this pressure for moulding the jaws, and the milk is obtained too easily, with resulting lack of stimulation for development. Another important point is the amount of trouble involved in bottle-feeding, the preparation of the milk formula, sterilization and preparation of the bottle and careful cleaning afterwards.

However, for one reason or another some mothers find it impossible to breast-feed and in that case the bottle will be an adequate substitute if it is carefully chosen and carefully looked after. There are now a number of well-designed feeding bottles available which do simulate the action of the breast. The mother must guard against being impatient and enlarging the hole in the rubber teat with a needle or pin to speed things up. The excuse usually is that baby is hungry or greedy and can't wait to get enough inside! Too easy sucking should be avoided. It may lead to 'tongue thrusting' and crooked jaws.

If the mother is taking fluoride herself almost none passes to the child in her milk and so if there is none or little in the water supply a fluoride supplement can be given to the child, starting at two or three weeks. The dose must be carefully worked out according to the amount in the public water supply, but this is an example of various doses:

Added fluoride dosage (milligrams per day)

Age	Concentration of fluoride in the drinking water (parts per million)		
	less than 0.3	0.3–0.7	0.7 & over
2 weeks – 2 years	0.25.	0.0 .	0.0.
2 – 3 years	0.50.	0.25.	0.0.
3 – 16 years	1.00.	0.50.	0.0.

Sodium fluoride tablets (2.2 mg) contain 1.0 mg of fluoride. Therefore the smallest dose indicated above is a quarter of a tablet.

It is better to ask your chemist for a fluoride liquid such as Luride Oral Paediatric Drops (Hoyt) which can be measured drop by drop much more accurately than trying to break a tablet into quarters. But, before doing anything, show the chart above to your dentist or doctor and get him to prescribe the correct dose for your area. See page 63 on Fluorides.

As your child gets older the teeth erupt and they should be cleaned by mother or another adult. Children under seven are not able to brush effectively, but it is useful training to let them try every day, handling the brush themselves and then the parent follows up to make sure a useful result has been obtained.

Dummies or comforters for babies are not as badly thought of as in years past. A baby will suck something, a thumb, blanket or comforter. If comforters are used: (1) they must be clean. (2) They must *not* be dipped in sugary substances. (3) They should not be of the 'miniature feeder' type which can have sugary fluids put in them. Blackcurrant syrups for babies and children are usually loaded with sugar and will rot the teeth as they form if left in contact with them.

A *child's* toothbrush should be used. This of course has a small head and a short handle. The handle should not have a pointed end. There is now a good choice of children's brushes made to British Standards BS 5757 (1979).

Use the smallest possible amount of a well known manufacturer's fluoride toothpaste. Do not use supermarket toothpastes (see section on Choosing a dentifrice). Use a small amount because young children swallow all sorts of things and swallowing soapy toothpaste can be unpleasant. A small fraction of the fluoride in a quarter-inch strip of toothpaste if swallowed will do no harm.

Why look after the baby teeth?

If the first teeth are allowed to decay they may be lost and as the first teeth keep the place for the developing permanent teeth, and because the gaps may close, the permanent teeth may be crowded out and there will be crooked teeth and the need for expensive and tedious orthodontic treatment. It might even mean the loss of some perfectly good second teeth because of the lack of room for them. It is possible for an infected baby tooth to affect the developing permanent tooth beneath. So you *must* look after the child's first teeth. If your child has unavoidably to lose a first tooth it is wise to discuss the fitting of a space retainer, often just a small metal bar, which keeps the space open for the second tooth to grow into when it's ready.

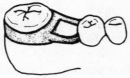

Figure 15. Space maintainer constructed of metal and fixed to the teeth to hold open the space for an erupting tooth.

The child's food

When the child is weaned, what food should be offered? Chemist's shops and supermarkets are full of jars of baby foods of all types, chicken and vegetable, banana and custard, etc. It is horrifying to note that almost all of these are loaded with sugar, or sweeteners. There may not be enough to do any harm to the teeth (although there probably is) but what does happen is that the child, because everything is sweet, develops a craving for sweet things. The answer is to buy a mincer and grind up fresh vegetables and small amounts of meat, sieve them and serve them to baby. It is possible for a child to grow up without developing a taste for sweet things, because it has never had any. But mothers can spoil everything by sweetening the baby's bottle.

Avoid: cola drinks which are sugar-loaded; blackcurrant syrup drinks; sugary breakfast foods, i.e. sugar-coated cereals and the like.

Children can be lazy and do not like to chew. That is why they prefer junk foods, fish fingers, baked beans, cakes, even hamburgers and chips – none of which requires much chewing. If parents encourage this attitude and do not give children food that needs chewing (like salads and hard vegetables) the teeth will deteriorate.

Finally if the child *must* have sweets it is better to have them all at once (at a mealtime) than spaced out through the day when the teeth will come under continuous attack.

When to start visits to the dentist

The ideal starting age for visiting the dentist is about two-and-a-half to three years. The advantages of an early start are:

1. Very few small children (with sensible parents) will have been exposed to anxiety arising from tales of dental 'horrors', especially from boasting or bloodthirsty schoolmates. It would be encouraging to believe that the public image of the dentist has changed completely, but regrettably, almost all newspaper articles, children's stories and other mass media outlets tend to concentrate on key emotive words such as toothache, drill, blood, extractions and 'pulling'. The child who becomes a friend of the practice before coming under this harmful influence will later reject the accounts of trauma as alien to itself and the practice it attends. Indeed, it becomes possible, when the child is older, to emphasize that early regular care is one factor which avoids the discomfort which may have been recounted to him by his schoolmates.

2. If the parent has been sensible about sweets and feeding-bottles there should be little or no decay. Hence very few small children will associate their own teeth with pain. The dentist may go on from this point maintaining a 'no-pain' approach for many years.

3. Attendance from pre-school age enhances the value of the dentist's preventive methods. There has been no time to acquire bad habits. Thus, the child grows up with dentistry and accepts it as the natural part of existence. At the time of the first visit at two-and-a-half to three years the primary teeth are all erupted through the gums and research has shown that this is the period when fluoride, when applied to the teeth by the dentist or hygienist, is taken up by the enamel most readily.

The dentist checks the teeth very carefully and then he or his hygienist will start to paint fluorides on the teeth. This is called topical fluoride and takes about fifteen to twenty minutes to go round the mouth in perhaps two or three-minute sections. There is no pain and the child usually enjoys the experience. The frequency of application varies but, because the intervals are convenient to remember, parents should take the children in during school holidays, i.e. every four months. This has cut down the amount of dental repair work required on the teeth. There are now thirty-year-olds who have had topical fluoride since the age of two-and-a-half and have never had a filling. The cost of topical treatments has been repaid many times over by the saving on other work. The dentist can reduce the number of topical treatments after sixteen to seventeen years.

4. If there is tooth decay starting it can be spotted early and treated with the minimum of discomfort.

Making the first appointment

The parent should preferably have taken the child a few times as an accompanying visitor while having his or her own dentistry. The dental staff will thus make friends with the child who will be shown around, perhaps being allowed to explore some of the more interesting gadgets. Whether the child will be seen by the parent's dentist or not (sometimes the parent's dentist does not attend children), when the first 'real' appointment is made, the secretary should be told that this will be the child's first dental appointment. Any other information regarding health, emotional problems, etc., should be mentioned. It is important to inquire whether the practice is a preventive one. It is likely to be so, but this was not the case up to ten years ago. If the practice is not heavily committed to the preventive approach, look for one that is.

Having made the appointment and before you go, tell your child about it without any anxieties. Let him know that the dentist is a friend who will help him to stay healthy and have beautiful teeth. The essence of success is to make the coming visit seem like an exciting adventure.

The pattern of the first visit

The first objective of the dentist or hygienist will be to make the visit a pleasant one and a great effort will be made to gain the child's confidence and trust. To start with, it may be possible to take X-rays if these are thought necessary. The panoramic X-ray film which is sometimes used shows all the teeth present and those still developing beneath the gums, and nothing is placed in the mouth. The X-ray radiation for panoramic films is very low. Such a film will show how the bones and teeth are growing.

The dental team will suggest to the parents, who should be present in the room at this time, that they too are part of 'the preventive team', and ways of preserving the child's dental health with a proper diet and the use of fluoride will be discussed. The way in which the teeth should be cleaned by the parent, and possibly the child, will be demonstrated. The mouth will be examined to make sure that everything is healthy, and any beginnings of decay will be noted and discussed and treatment will be arranged.

If the child, for some reason or other, is very nervous, or if he or she is under two years old, it may be necessary for the mother to hold the child in her lap while she herself is in the chair.

For a good start in dental life for your child:

1. Make the visits a fun trip.

2. Do not bribe your child to attend, or threaten the visit as a punishment.

3. Do not appear to be anxious about the visit yourself, and never say, 'it will not hurt'. That is the worst possible approach.

4. Do not wait until your child has toothache before taking him or her to the dentist.

5. Do not allow others to relate 'horror' stories to your child. After the first visit be prepared, depending on the dentist's or hygienist's instructions, to allow your child to enter the treatment room alone. Remember that treatment of the first (primary) teeth is important: to enable your child to chew satisfactorily; to keep the space for the permanent teeth waiting to come through from underneath; and to help speech.

6. Avoid tetracycline antibiotics for the infant, if possible. Otherwise teeth might become discoloured.

Cleft lip and cleft palate

It is a distressing experience for the mother to see her new baby with a cleft lip and palate. Such a deformity is very obvious, and often the parents have a feeling of guilt or shame. Defects in formation in which the two halves of the palate and lip fail to unite occur once in approximately 750 births. It would be reassuring for the parents to know just how much can be done to remedy the condition. Surgical treatment to close the lip defect is made early – often before the child leaves hospital with its mother for the first time. This is, of course, a good psychological factor for the mother and for other members of the family, and lessens the risk of 'rejection' of the child as not quite belonging. However, the time of surgery and its nature depends on the condition of the child – a decision to be made by the surgeon. The immediate problem at birth is that of feeding, and lip closure surgery helps this. Satisfactory treatment of the cleft palate/lip child requires a team effort and may involve all or any of the following: family doctor, paediatrician, dentist, orthodontist, prosthetist, oral surgeon, ENT surgeon, community service, plastic surgeon, speech therapist, dental technician and dental hygienist.

An appliance is necessary in a large proportion of cases to close the defect in the palate and this may be constructed in the form of a partial denture attached to the teeth. Often the teeth are displaced and may be so malaligned that they are difficult to clean and could easily decay. It is essential that careful preventive measures for preservation of the teeth are observed so that tooth loss is avoided. These teeth, whether first teeth or second, are needed for retention and support of the obturator which aids speech. Regular visits to the dentist and hygienist for plaque control and applications of fluoride are essential.

Of the one in 750 births where cleft palate occurs, some are due to genetic factors and others may be due to environmental accidents such as the taking of certain drugs during pregnancy or other outside influences. After such a birth the family doctor and the parents should investigate whether there is any genetic defect and, if so, consider whether they should risk further pregnancies.

The handicapped child

If your child is handicapped in some way you must mention it to the dentist and special care will be taken. Dental hygienists are trained to care for children with different handicaps and they will explain to the parent any special home dental care that is required.

The practice may also demonstrate individually designed brushes or holders for those who have difficulty in gripping ordinary brushes. If your general dentist is not able to attend to handicapped children or even normal children for one reason or another, or if he believes your child is a 'special' case requiring specialist treatment, he may refer you to a *paedodontist* who is a specialist in children's dentistry. This may be at the local hospital or nearest dental teaching hospital or could be arranged privately.

Orthodontics

If your child has an irregular jaw formation or lack of room for all the teeth your dentist will advise you at the correct time about the treatment that will be required. He may be able to do the necessary correction himself but many general dentists will refer you to an *orthodontist* – a specialist in the regulation (straightening) of teeth (mostly of children, although orthodontists now straighten the teeth of adults when this is considered feasible). See Chapter 16, Cosmetic Dentistry.

Malocclusion. An irregular jaw or crooked teeth may be inherited. One well-documented example is the Habsburg jaw which was a dominant feature in the Spanish royal family of the Habsburgs, with the enormously protruded lower jaw. Macaulay wrote of Charles II of Spain, 'the malformation of the jaw characteristic of this family is so serious that he could not masticate his food.' Some children grow with jaws that are too small to accommodate their teeth which become crowded and crooked. The normal arrangement of the jaws and the way they should meet is shown in Figure 1.

Acquired defects. Malformations of growth can be acquired by sucking and pulling on poorly designed artificial nipples in feeding bottles or the lack of stimulation caused by too easy feeding from bottles where the hole has been enlarged. Other deformities can occur by thumb- or finger-sucking if continued past the age of five or six. The forward projection of the top front teeth and backward inclination of the lower front teeth caused by thumb-sucking often corrects itself if the habit is stopped early. All too often thumb-sucking is a sign of anxiety; therefore do not increase the anxiety by threats. Kindness, consideration, advice and help from the

dentist will usually solve the problem. Another cause of malformation is the habit of tongue-thrusting through the front teeth.
This leads to a gap between these teeth. The tongue-thrusting
habit is difficult to correct. Too early loss of the primary teeth due
to decay will allow the remaining teeth to close up and there will be
no room for the succeeding teeth to come through into the correct
position. Thus the parent can be involved in preventing much
malocclusion by seeing that the primary teeth are cared for and are
retained until the second teeth are ready to erupt. However, if a
primary tooth is, through some misfortune, unsavable the dentist
will consider the necessity of inserting the space maintainer
previously mentioned. Trouble can be caused by mouth breathing
and it is then wise to have the nasal passages checked –
occasionally adenoids can almost block them.

With regular attendance at the dentist any over-prolonged
habits, such as thumb-sucking or other tendency to push the teeth
out of alignment, will be carefully watched and the time for
interception to prevent deformity will be decided by the dentist,
who may then construct a simple appliance or refer to an orthodontist. Sometimes a simple remedy for a crowded mouth may be
the extraction of a permanent tooth or teeth in order to make
room. Parents are sometimes horrified that a dentist has
recommended the loss of four permanent (and good!) teeth in
order to correct a crowded mouth. The reason for four teeth is that
by removing one tooth from each quadrant of the mouth, upper
right and left, lower right and left, there is an even amount of
space created all round the mouth. Otherwise, if space is created
on one side of the mouth only, the teeth may be spaced out on that
side and there is a danger that the front teeth will be off-centre.
The consideration of malocclusion and crooked teeth is a very
individual one and depends on careful assessment and knowledge
by the dentist, but the regular attendance and concern of the
parents is most important. Neglect of the dentist's advice at the
stage when simple treatment will suffice may condemn the child to
much more difficult treatment with appliances at a later time. It is
difficult to understand the attitude of some parents. Not long ago a
dentist told one mother that her son required orthodontic
treatment because his upper teeth jutted out rabbit wise, and it was
time something was done about it. The lady decided that she did

not want any straightening of her son's teeth. Reason? 'I think he looks cute like that – just like a bunny!' Will her 'bunny' be grateful to her when he is called that by his colleagues at university or place of work?

If your child needs to attend for orthodontic advice your dentist may refer him or her to a specialist orthodontist at a dental hospital or one of the specialized orthodontic departments in various parts of the country, or you may decide to have a private consultation with an orthodontist.

The first consultation will consist of a very thorough examination with impressions taken for the construction of models of the mouth and jaws for study by the dentist. X-rays and facial profile registration may also be taken. A great deal of planning will be done before treatment (if required) is started. The orthodontist may also delay the treatment until the correct time. This may be governed by the state of eruption of the teeth. Many different appliances are constructed for different conditions. Some appliances are fixed to the teeth so that the wires and springs which guide the teeth into the correct positions are attached and are removable only by the dentist. This has certain advantages which the dentist will explain if he considers such a fixture necessary.

Modern improvements have almost eliminated the unsightly banding of the teeth and many of the attachments (brackets), often transparent, which hold the wires are directly bonded to the enamel with the new remarkable adhesive techniques. One disadvantage is that very careful cleaning by the young wearer is imperative because food and plaque are easily trapped in all this apparatus which cannot be removed for cleaning. Special small brushes are provided for this purpose. A careful check must be kept by the parent on this cleaning, otherwise the risk of decay or

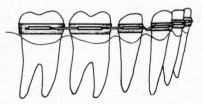

Figure 16. Fixed orthodontic bands and wires.

gum disease is very high. Fixed appliances have many advantages however: treatment is more certain and cannot easily be upset by the patient 'forgetting' to wear his or her plate.

Other appliances are removable and thus more readily cleansable. Removable appliances are not always so certain in their action because of the possibility that they may not be worn or may be lost or broken, sometimes by being sat on! There are other treatments which may involve wearing a headcap, with wires gently pulling on the jaws to alter their relative positions.

The orthodontist will discuss his proposals when he has made up his treatment plan and outlined it, often in writing. The family dentist may be able to explain more about the treatment when he is seen for regular check-ups. Parents may not understand that orthodontists do not repair teeth and thus they omit visits to the family dentist, sometimes with disastrous results. The parents' influence must be very positive when orthodontic treatment is started because the young adolescent, principally for social reasons, may not want to continue wearing appliances. Encouragement by a parent with the help of instructional and educational material obtainable either from the dentist or orthodontist is an important feature of success in orthodontic treatment.

Foods to avoid while wearing orthodontic appliances

Very hard foods may bend or break the delicate tubes or wires of the orthodontic appliances which are fixed to the teeth. Sticky foods, e.g. toffee, may loosen the bands and attach to the wires and teeth. Avoid sweets, chewing gum, hard nuts, hard rolls, etc.

14
Restoring Teeth

Fillings

A tooth may become damaged and a part of it lost. The major reason for this is dental decay, although occasionally accidental breakage occurs. If a great deal of the tooth has been destroyed (and usually much more decay is present inside the tooth than appears to the outside view) a crown may be required which would cover all or nearly all the tooth, holding the remaining parts together and restoring the complete shape.

Silver amalgam

For the usual type of cavity the most commonly used material is silver amalgam which is about seventy per cent silver alloyed with other materials such as tin, copper, etc., to a very exact formula in order to give the filling maximum desirable properties. This alloy of silver is used by the dentist either in the form of a fine powder or as pellets (the same powder compressed into little pills) and is mixed just before use with a precise amount of mercury, usually in a vibratory machine called an amalgamator, and the resulting putty-like mass is packed into the prepared cavity in the tooth and sets hard in a few hours. The hardening time varies with the different makes of amalgam alloys and may be from a few minutes to a few hours. There are a number of new (and very expensive) alloys which achieve a rapid hard set. Many of these now cost the dentist as much or more than the basic price of gold five or six years ago.

Silver amalgam has a number of good qualities. For small fillings in areas which are not too visible from the front it is ideal and it also has a built-in protective action which tends to discourage further decay. However, it is a brittle material and will break if extended too far as in a large cavity and also the poor colour (even when highly polished) does not make it usable in front teeth. Silver amalgam tends to *expand* very slightly with time and on occasion, if the remaining tooth surrounding an amalgam filling is fragile or thin, the outer shell or wall can be fractured off. A 'crown' enveloping the remainder of the tooth would be the ideal restoration in that case, but if this is not possible – perhaps because of its high cost – an alternative may be tried. Tiny stainless steel or other non-corrodible threaded metal pins are cemented or screwed into channels which are drilled into the inside of the tooth – to about 2mm in depth. These pins form a framework around which the silver amalgam is packed and held quite securely. Even if a crown is going to be made eventually it is often necessary to build up the shape of the tooth with amalgam in the same way, using pins.

Preparation of the tooth for amalgam

Before any filling is inserted the dentist must be sure that all the decay has been removed from all parts of the cavity. In order to do this he will use the dental 'drill' (the modern high speed drill with water spray) in order to cut back the walls of the tooth around the decay so that there are no ledges under which decay can exist and be missed by him. All this may be done while the tooth is rendered painless by a local injection of anaesthetic solution. The tooth

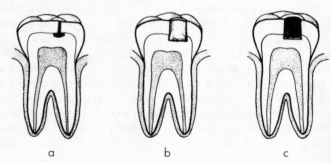

a　　　　　　b　　　　　　c

Figure 17. Stages of filling with amalgam. (a) The decay penetrates the enamel to the dentine. (b) The cavity is prepared and (c) the silver amalgam is inserted. Note the thin protective lining below the amalgam.

structure is softened by the decay process and this soft material is scooped out with sharp instruments (excavators) which are like tiny sharp spoons.

Another task is to remove all weak edges of the cavity because these may chip off during eating after the filling has been inserted, leaving a gap which can cause further decay. When all these edges have been smoothed off there are a number of other finishing touches before filling. Amalgam has no adhesive properties and if it is going to be used it must be locked into the tooth by so shaping the cavity (wider at the bottom than at the surface) that the filling once set cannot fall out. It is also necessary to protect the pulp inside the tooth because a metal filling may exert pressure on the underlying nerve when chewing and it will also conduct a temperature change. Therefore the dentist paints in or places a lining of a paste which just covers the bottom of the cavity and usually has a sedative action on the pulp below the floor of the cavity.

When one or more side walls of the tooth have been lost, a thin steel band (a matrix band) is placed around the tooth. This will aid in the correct shaping of the filling and will avoid excess filling being pushed into the gum which would lead to inflammation. The amalgam filling is then packed very tightly into the cavity, and when this has been completely filled the dentist carves the surface of the amalgam level with the natural tooth surface and smooths it off. Eventually the amalgam filling, like all fillings, requires polishing, but this is not done for at least forty-eight hours. An amalgam filling is not at its best unless it is polished, otherwise the slightly roughened surface can pick up bacteria and favour breakdown at the edges. The patient should not mind attending for a short visit so that all the fillings can be polished.

Tooth-coloured fillings

Metal fillings either of silver amalgam or gold look unsightly in the front of the mouth so fillings which match the tooth were developed and new ones are still being introduced. There is no wholly satisfactory tooth-coloured filling material and the ones which are available are for the front teeth and should not be used in the back of the mouth where they would be involved in chewing. This type of tooth-coloured filling will not stand up to the wear and tear of chewing. Patients often demand these fillings for molar teeth and until recently the dentist was correct in explaining that we have no tooth-coloured material with sufficient resistance to chewing action. With the present rapid development of new materials it should be possible to fill some back teeth with the newer fillings. However, the only way in which any extensive loss of tooth tissue in back teeth can be restored to look like natural teeth is at present by preparing the tooth (which means grinding away the outside layer) and rebuilding with a gold shell on which a complete covering of tooth-coloured porcelain is bonded by expert technicians in their laboratories. Such work is of course expensive and time-consuming.

Tooth-coloured fillings for cavities in front teeth used to be made of a cement-like material – silicate cement. This discoloured rapidly in some mouths, and the surface dissolved fairly quickly, especially in acid mouths. Today most dentists use *composite* fillings which are basically a resin filled with tiny particles of quartz for strength. Usually the filling is mixed from two pastes with the resultant single paste packed into the prepared cavity, setting in two or three minutes. These fillings are very hard and can be made to adhere very closely to enamel by etching the surface of the enamel for a minute or so with a special weak acid which opens up thousands of pores into which the resin enters and becomes locked to the enamel surface. In this way it often happens that, provided all decay is removed, comparatively little drilling is necessary to retain the filling.

Other composite filling materials consist of a single paste which is placed in position in the cavity, shaped correctly and caused to set by the influence of a special lamp giving out light similar to the range of ultra-violet light. The newer lamps use special projector bulbs and are quite safe. Although not a perfect material – leakage between the filling and the tooth still takes place as with other materials, and obtaining a good polished surface is difficult – these composite filling materials have made a great difference to the ease with which a good appearance can be restored to the front teeth and many hitherto complicated restorative procedures have been made much easier. But it must be borne in mind that none of these materials is 'permanent' and in certain areas and conditions must be renewed or 'topped up' at intervals which vary according to the amount of wear and exposure to which each one is subjected. Even with these improved posterior 'cosmetic fillings' it would not be sensible to try to persuade your dentist to substitute these for sound metal fillings already in place.

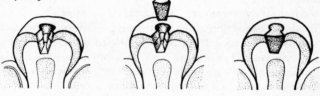

Figure 18. (a) Cavity prepared for a gold inlay. (b) The inlay, which is cast from a wax pattern of the cavity. (c) The inlay cemented into place.

Gold fillings

These are usually in the form of *inlays* and although non-precious metals have been used, there is really nothing quite as satisfactory as gold. The dentist needs to take a pattern of the cavity which must have no retentive undercuts (see Silver amalgam) but the shape must be such that the opening is slightly wider at the surface than at the bottom of the cavity. An impression must be taken of the cavity as the gold inlay is made in the laboratory. At least two visits will be necessary. Inlays have many advantages. Because they are cast in one piece they are virtually unbreakable, and large areas of decayed teeth can thus be restored. They can be polished to a high lustre and the edges can be burnished over the join with the tooth virtually sealing out bacteria. Many patients ask: 'Isn't gold too soft to be used as a filling material?' In fact dentists use special golds which are scientifically prepared with added materials such as platinum, copper, silver, etc., and so different strengths can be achieved for different purposes. The melting point of the gold can be varied so that, for example, some special golds can be made to remain solid while porcelain is fused on to them. The usual golds used for inlays would have melted before the porcelain could become attached. The development of such special golds means that you cannot take your mother's old gold ring to the dentist and ask him to use it for your next inlay. The technician needs to use the specially prepared golds for exact castings. It also means that the gold the dentist uses costs even more than the current astronomical gold prices quoted in the daily newspapers.

The present extraordinary rise in gold costs is causing concern to dentists and technicians because there is still no substitute for this metal for many of the exacting procedures in restorative dentistry.

Gold has many advantages in its adaptability to casting, shaping and its ability accurately to fit with great precision. Disadvantages are its colour, varying from light yellow to orange according to composition and, of course, its cost. It is often possible to make a window in the more noticeable area and cover this with replaceable tooth-coloured material as long as it is not on the chewing surface of the tooth.

When the inlay has been cast, polished and tried in the mouth it is cemented into place with a special cement.

Comparison of fillings

The universal posterior filling is still *silver amalgam* but, as shown above, it has its limitations.

Gold is a first-class material but it needs first-class technique. It can be said that a gold inlay which is a lot less than perfect is much worse than a similar amalgam filling. If you have a first-class dentist – and can afford it – have gold inlays in your back teeth where they don't show too much. Beware, however, of mixing gold and amalgam in different parts of the mouth. The fear used to be of what is called 'galvanism', i.e. currents (which could cause minor shocks to the teeth – not dangerous but annoying) when two metals of different materials touched momentarily.

Some dentists are against the mixing of materials as fillings because the differences in wear may cause an imbalance in the way the jaws mesh and may give rise to joint problems.

Tooth-coloured materials have already been described (page 120).

One other type of filling may be mentioned in passing – the *gold foil* filling. This is of pure gold in cohesive leaf form and it can be beaten into the prepared cavity by tiny increments which weld to each other. The process is time-consuming, requires considerable skill and is now rarely done in Britain. There are pockets of enthusiasts in the United States, especially on the north-west coast, who use gold foil and produce excellent results. Many gold foil fillings have lasted for fifty years or more and still look as good as new.

Regrettably we must look upon these in general as a past luxury for the vast majority of patients, especially as their use is restricted mainly to small cavities.

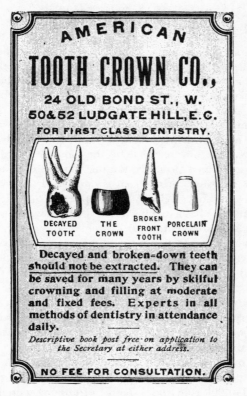

Figure 19. Crowning teeth is not new! Advertisement, *c.* 1897. (*Mary Evans Picture Library*)

Gold crowns

The posterior teeth are sometimes so broken down that they have to be rebuilt and are covered for complete protection by a cast gold crown. Occasionally, if the patient is over-conscious that the gold shows, the visible parts can be obscured by tooth-coloured plastic material, or for complete natural tooth simulation a bonded gold-porcelain crown can be constructed. This latter is the most expensive of the alternatives mentioned (see Chapter 16, Cosmetic Dentistry).

The dental drill

Drilling is really a misnomer. Teeth are usually not drilled using the tip of the tool as one would use a power drill to make holes in the wall. The modern, very small cutting tools (called burs) coated with fine diamonds or made with tiny tungsten carbide blades along their sides, revolve at enormous speeds (about 250,000 to 350,000 rpm) and the sides grind away the edges of already established holes widening them so that the underlying decay becomes accessible for removal by the dentist. In this way the cavity is also shaped properly for the filling. The stem of the diamond or tungsten carbide tool is only about 1mm thick and about 2cm long. It is held in a handpiece about the size of a fountain pen. This has a turbine inside the head which is driven by compressed air and gives the bur its tremendous speed. The effect of this is a very gentle action because there is very little power (or torque) generated and the dentist could easily prevent the bur from rotating by holding it with his fingers (before it starts to rotate!). He cannot exert pressure on the tooth with the bur but must remove tooth substance by movement as if he were painting the tooth. The speed of the drill smooths out the action so that very little vibration is felt because each blade touches the tooth for a minute fraction of a second.

The fear of the drill arose from the older 'conventional' motor-driven equipment where the heavier-stemmed bur revolved at about 4,000–6,000 rpm and a degree of force was applied to the tooth in order to obtain any cutting action. The original tools were made of simple steel and blunted rapidly on touching the tooth enamel which is an extremely hard, glasslike substance. Thus, preparing a cavity was a noisy, prolonged and unpleasant sensation whether pain was felt or not. Another modern improvement is the accompanying water spray on the bur tip while rotating. This was necessary because the high speed generates considerable heat and therefore tooth tissue or the pulp could be damaged by overheating. The cooling effect also enables small increments of 'drilling' to be carried out, often without anaesthetic, because much of the painful grinding of the 'old days' was the result of overheating the tooth, even at the low speeds employed.

Of course, there are still grounds for complaint, although minor ones. The high-pitched noise of the turbine can be objectionable, but even this has been modified in recent years. The dentist who has his ears assaulted by the noise all day and every day may sometimes find that his hearing is affected, but certainly the patient, for the short time of exposure, suffers no ill effects in this way. Another requirement, because of the high volume of water used in the cooling system, is an efficient water suction system. Inevitably this led to the introduction of '*four-handed*' *dentistry* in which the dentist is helped at the chairside by an assistant who has the important duty to see that no water collects in the mouth.

There are many different types of cutting aids with different shapes depending on the job to be done, whether it be preparing the cavity for silver amalgam or a gold inlay, or reducing the whole enamel around the tooth for a crown. The dentist will also use hand cutting instruments, tiny sharp chisels to chip or smooth off edges and will scoop out decay with tiny, sharp, spoon-like excavators.

The old type of drill has not been eliminated. It is still very important, because of its precision bearings, in cutting tiny straight channels (about 2mm) and also where slow action is required such as polishing the teeth or fillings with small brushes or rubber polishers.

With the use of practically painless injections rendering the tooth completely insensitive and the modern, smooth, rotor-driven, high-speed bur there can no longer be fear of 'the drill' and anyone who continues to worry about it has not experienced today's dentistry.

15
Root Canal Treatment (Endodontics)

Some patients are terrified if they are told that, 'the nerve of the tooth has to be removed.' I explained in the early part of this book that the pulp is composed of nerve tissue, blood vessels, protective cells and other materials. This supplies sensation to the tooth and also nourishment to the dentine and enables it to be repaired.

Dental decay may extend so far into the tooth that bacteria reach the pulp and it becomes inflamed and painful. If the decay is treated in time the inflammation, if mild, may be reversed and the pulp may recover. However, the pulp may become so damaged that the only alternatives are its removal or the removal of the tooth.

Sometimes the pulp dies slowly and quietly on its own, perhaps after an injury (a hit on the front tooth of a child) and, if left alone, the dead elements in the pulp putrefy and leak through the apex (the tip of the root) into the bone and either a chronic or acute abscess results.

There are other reasons why root canal treatment is judged necessary by the dentist – perhaps for cosmetic reasons when making a crown. The dentist will discuss this with the patient. If he feels that the type of root canal treatment requires the attention of a specialist he will refer the case to an *endodontist*.

The pulps of front teeth are easier to treat than those at the back of the mouth. The incisors and canines have one root and therefore usually only a single root canal. The molars usually have three canals in each tooth and, because of their position, root canal treatment presents problems for the dentist. This is particularly so if the patient is middle-aged or older, as the canals become finer with age. With present-day local anaesthetic techniques, removal of the pulp is a painless procedure and the dentist accomplishes it with very fine instruments which clean out the canals inside the roots almost to their tips. He uses progressively larger file-like instruments until he is convinced that the canals are clean.

All this is usually done with a rubber mask around the tooth (called a *rubber dam*) which is placed around the tooth with a special clamp. This is necessary to exclude saliva which may infect the inside of the canals. The dam also ensures that instruments and other materials do not drop into the mouth where they may be swallowed if the patient makes a sudden movement. Once the root canals are thoroughly cleaned they are washed out by special solutions. The whole procedure may require a number of sessions of delicate work. Root canals cannot be left empty since bacteria may get in and reinfect them. The entire canal is usually sealed with special (sometimes antiseptic) sealing agents and such root canal fillers as gutta percha or silver points. The dentist will take X-rays at various stages and check that his work is meticulously accurate. Once he is convinced that the canal or canals are satisfactorily sealed he can proceed with his planned filling or crowning of the tooth.

Because of the precision and skill required for such work the speciality of endodontics is a very lucrative one in the United States and the endodontists there probably earn the highest fees of any speciality in dentistry. However, the treatment can be costly to the dentist himself. Many of the fine needle-like files can only be used once and are discarded. Most of these are made abroad and sometimes ten are used in the treatment of one tooth. But the alternative procedure of extracting the tooth means the eventual further cost of constructing a replacement such as a bridge or denture which can be more expensive than saving the tooth by endodontic treatment.

Sometimes a tooth such as an upper incisor develops an acute abscess and becomes very painful and there is swelling in the jaw above the tooth and throbbing. In such a case the pulp of the tooth is 'dead'. The dentist will make a hole with a diamond 'drill' though the back of the tooth (a local anaesthetic injection is usually not needed) and will reach the pulp chamber. Pus from the abscess will start to drain from the tooth and almost immediate relief will be felt. Subsequently the dentist goes through the above-mentioned routine of root canal treatment and eventually fills up the hole he made in the back of the tooth.

At the completion of such treatment the tooth crown often has been so destroyed by decay or for other reasons that an *artificial crown* will be required. Because the interior of the tooth, including the roots, has been hollowed out in the cleansing of the canals there is a tendency to weakness and fracture. This is rather like the possibility of a dead tree trunk snapping off. Therefore the roots are reinforced with an interior steel or cast gold post to which a new crown is attached.

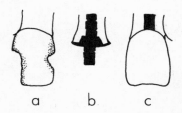

Figure 20. Post Crown. (a) Shows a much decayed tooth. (b) The root canal has been filled and a metal post fitted. (c) A crown is fitted to the post.

Occasionally, it may be impossible to clean out the root canal and seal it by the methods described above and therefore the dentist may carry out an operation called an apicectomy in which he opens up the gum above the tooth (under local anaesthetic, usually), cleans out any infected matter around the apex and seals the tip of the root with some material such as amalgam. The gum is stitched back into place and healing usually occurs in three to four days.

16
Cosmetic Dentistry

Perhaps the reader turned to this section first because, worried about unsightly teeth, he or she hoped that here would be revealed the secret of a beautiful smile. The truth is that the term 'cosmetic dentistry' was probably coined by the press or popular magazines. It would be difficult to find any university dental school which offered a course in 'dental cosmetics'. In fact *all* dental treatment should take into account the necessity either to maintain or improve the appearance. A separate speciality of 'cosmetic dentistry', which we understand to mean making the mouth and smile attractive, should not exist. However, mouths may be made healthy by fillings and the gums treated by surgery, but the patient may be dissatisfied with the appearance. We all know how television discloses unsightly teeth in performers and how distracting this can be. Therefore, apart from the usual repair of the teeth, people sometimes ask for special attention to what they consider to be ugly teeth. The front teeth of course are the most obvious and it is these (six uppers and six lowers) which usually receive the most 'cosmetic attention'. We have mentioned in Chapter 14 that front teeth can be filled with materials which closely match the shade of the teeth. However, few fillings last for ever and eventually the tooth-coloured fillings wear or discolour slightly and need replacing. Frequent replacement of many of these in the same tooth may eventually weaken the tooth, necessitating a more drastic repair. A complete coverage by a veneer crown not only restores the whole tooth, but holds it together.

The porcelain crown

To construct a new crown for a tooth the enamel is removed by skimming it away with fast-moving diamond or tungsten carbide points, usually while the tooth is anaesthetized with a local injection. The stump of the crown is carefully shaped and impressions are taken to a millimetre below the gum line. A temporary (plastic) crown is fitted while a porcelain crown is constructed by the technician in the laboratory to the exact shade

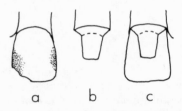

Figure 21. Construction and fitting of a porcelain jacket crown.

which the dentist has matched at the chairside. At the next appointment if both dentist and patient are satisfied as to the shape and colour, the crown is cemented into place with a special dental cement. The porcelain material is brittle in thin sections, but in recent years has been greatly strengthened by the addition of an aluminous core. The aluminous core is central to the crown and does not show at the front. Thus excellent colour matching is possible. Where there is so much impact from the opposing teeth on to the crown that even this reinforced porcelain is not strong enough, a special porcelain bonded to gold is used. The gold is either completely covered by the porcelain or some gold is left uncovered at the back of the crown to take the impact from the opposing teeth.

In either case it is possible for the dentist and technician to achieve excellent colour matches although obviously the life-like translucency obtained with the porcelain crown without gold is somewhat lacking. A disadvantage of the latter crown, because of the gold in it (and it is highly specialized gold with platinum and other metals), is the high cost. This is balanced somewhat by the fact that the gold/porcelain crown is virtually indestructible and does not tarnish or lose its matching colour.

A single tooth or group of teeth may require crowning. The following conditions require crowns:

1. Discolouration of a tooth or teeth.

2. Misshapen or malformed teeth, and front teeth which have been damaged by lemon or grapefruit juice in excess.

3. Groups of teeth which are badly aligned.

4. Groups of teeth crowned to make room for another tooth slightly out of line.

5. A missing tooth, which may be replaced by crowning the teeth either side of the gap with a false crown joined to these. This is a fixed bridge.

6. A natural space between two teeth, e.g. as in a gap between the two front incisors.

7. Front teeth which project forwards or are splayed out and, conversely, front teeth which are set back too far.

There are innumerable variations. No two mouths are alike, neither will two jacket crown preparations be the same. Every crown must be individually constructed in a meticulous and painstaking fashion.

Where there are overlapping teeth in the front because of shortage of space it may be possible to prepare a number of teeth (often one or two more than seem to be involved in the crowding) for crowns. The final crowns are each made narrower than the natural teeth thus giving sufficient room to align them in a pleasing manner. However, if one or two teeth are grossly out of line the roots and the prepared stumps may be so far away from the arch of the adjoining teeth that it may be necessary to remove the pulp from the root: see Chapter 15. A metal post is then inserted into the root; this will carry an artificial stump preparation which can be constructed at such an angle that it lines up with the other teeth. This is a 'post crown'. See Fig. 2.

I cannot here discuss all the possibilities for crowns. However, bear in mind that there must always be careful planning before any such reconstruction work is commenced.

The dentist will take impressions of the teeth in both jaws and mount the casts from these in correct relationship to each other. You can ask to see a 'mock up', i.e. a remodelled version of your mouth as the dentist plans it on completion. It enables you to decide whether the expected result makes the complicated and expensive constructions worthwhile. Having agreed to the plan, the next step is to arrange for an estimate.

The dentist may refer the patient to someone who is more expert in such work, but in all cases the following investigations must be carried out:

1. The general health of the patient must be ascertained, together with his or her ability to tolerate long sessions in the dental chair, if necessary.

2. Radiographs must be taken of all the teeth involved; the state of the dental pulp must be checked.

3. Models of the mouth must be prepared.

4. Colour photographs of the condition should be taken. In this respect you may gain confidence from the dentist's previous successes by asking to see 'before and after' photographs or slides of other similarly treated cases.

Colour matching

Some people believe that if they are going to have most of the front teeth crowned (or as some newspapers call it, 'capped'), they might as well have them much lighter in shade, even *white*. But there are no natural white teeth. Even the lightest youthful teeth are made up of shades of yellow with other shades such as blue (at the tips) and some grey. A piece of white card cut into a strip and placed along the front teeth will show you how absurd a really white set of teeth will look.

As people age, the teeth darken slightly and you should therefore take the advice of your dentist (and also that of the technician) on the correct shade of crown for your facial colour and the match for any other adjacent teeth. It is important to be certain about the choice of colour because once porcelain teeth have been fired especially for you to the stated shade, the only way to change it is to start again. All sorts of staining which are natural to the teeth at different ages can be built into the finished porcelain crown. It makes for an excellent natural appearance if the dentist and technician build slight imperfections into the enamel. In this way the too-perfect crown, which looks artificial, can be avoided.

Shapes of crowns

Do not expect all the teeth to be even and the same size, shape and length. Some patients bring along a fashion magazine and show the teeth of the cover girl, not realizing that artist's touched-up teeth may look all right on the cover, but in real life will look ridiculous. As some of the people who ask for teeth 'like the [twenty-year-old] girl on the cover' are middle-aged ladies, one could reply, 'If you can wear her clothes as she does, you might be able to have the same teeth!' Teeth grow in many shapes and forms. Usually the line of the teeth looks better if slightly broken up. The upper lateral incisors (second from the front on each side) should be narrower and slightly shorter than the two larger central incisors. There should also be a slight tilt of the long axis of the teeth slightly towards the centre line of the face. That is, teeth do not grow straight up and down like this,

$$| \; | \; | \; |$$

but tilt a little like this,

$$\backslash \; \backslash \; / \; /$$

Again, you must trust the dentist's judgement about choosing the right shape and size of teeth. If there is doubt the dentist may make a preliminary crown in tooth-coloured plastic and allow the patient to wear it for a week or so. It can then be adjusted easily according to comments. Once the plastic shapes are to the patient's satisfaction the dentist can copy them and finish in porcelain. Of course this may add slightly to the expense but it does ensure a happier result in the end.

It is often necessary to improve the appearance of back teeth, which have to be crowned. This is more important in lower teeth because the tops of these show much more obviously than upper back teeth. A bonded porcelain to gold crown is often made for lower teeth. This has an inner core of gold to which is fired a complete porcelain covering matching the colour of the adjacent teeth. It would not be possible to construct the chewing surface of back teeth of porcelain only because the forces of mastication would soon cause a fracture. Similarly, missing teeth are replaced by using bonded gold porcelain crowns so that the finished result is a series of units which resemble natural teeth and are not removable.

Whole mouth reconstruction

Cosmetic dentistry does not consist only of crown construction. It may not always be possible to correct gross abnormalities by crowning alone. Also, it may not be necessary. It is better if crowning can be avoided because it involves removal of large amounts of the outer structure of the tooth.

Most people who believe they need 'cosmetic dentistry' are concerned with the appearance of front teeth. Very often the poor character of these front teeth may be due to the loss or wearing away of the back (molar and premolar) teeth so that the jaws overclose (in extreme cases the chin can be brought up to the nose). There is less room for the upper and lower front teeth as a result. The back teeth meeting normally prevents overclosure. In cases of overclosure the front teeth may wear down until they are very short indeed and unsightly or they may fracture or, worse still, if the supporting jawbone is weak the teeth will splay out and loosen. Thus the dentist may, in his discussion about treatment, try to explain, 'yes, I know you have come to me about having nice-looking front teeth, but I cannot get a long-term successful result unless I build up the lost height at the back of your jaws.' This may mean (a) bridgework at the back of the mouth (or even partial dentures) to supply missing teeth, (b) crowning teeth which have worn down, (c) fitting onlays – gold caps which are cemented on to the prepared tops of the teeth.

In this way room is allowed for crowns of normal length and shape in the front, which look natural and, more important, which will last, with the teeth, for a long time. I mention this because when fees are discussed you may be horrified to find that so much extra cost is involved in doing something which was not envisaged when the request for 'nice-looking' front teeth was made. But if repairs at the back of the mouth are necessary it would be foolhardy to ignore the dentist's advice. You'll be throwing away good money and hours of sitting in the chair for an unsatisfactory final result, and you'll end up with a bad relationship with your dentist caused by frequent loss of those front crowns or teeth.

Cosmetic dentistry may be much more expensive than you expect. On the other hand, you may be pleasantly surprised that what looked to you like an 'impossible' situation can be corrected quite reasonably. And you may want to try out (but beware of the limitations) the short-term corrections mentioned in this section, which the dentist may carry out just to give you an idea how much better you will look, and which often last for many months or even years.

Charges may vary among dentists according to their standing and the location of their practice. Obviously in the centre of a city rents and other expenses – salaries, etc. – are high. Materials used are enormously costly and dentists may spend considerable sums travelling to dental conferences and post-graduate lectures all over the world to gain experience of the latest techniques and materials. Congress and convention organizers know that dentists are the greatest attenders of meetings and courses. The annual international dentist congress (FDI) may attract as many as 20,000 participants from all over the world. The costs of fees for *good* work should therefore be readily appreciated.

Orthodontics

Sometimes it may be possible, even in the adult, to move teeth into a more attractive position by the use of springs and wires. This work is undertaken by the orthodontist who generally straightens children's teeth. The appliance may not look attractive but many of the present-day orthodontic appliances are reasonably unobtrusive and some may be worn at night only.

Surgery

For gross deformities not correctable by other means, surgical treatment can be arranged. Surgery is recommended for such conditions as the grossly enlarged lower jaw (the Habsburg jaw) or too small, underslung jaws. The operation consists of taking a section of jaw bone away on either side, pushing the chin back and wiring the ends together (done from an incision which later becomes almost invisible), or the jaw is split across from the inside (like splitting a £5 note) and the two sides of the split are slid on each other either back for the too prominent jaw, or forward for the underslung jaw. The jaws are then immobilized for some weeks with splints.

The success rate is very high, but the operation must be carried out by an expert! Usually in this condition it is best to attend a dental teaching hospital for advice. It may be necessary to combine all three approaches, i.e. surgery, orthodontics and crowning in order to obtain an excellent cosmetic result. Because the jaws are wired together for some weeks after surgery, eating is difficult.

Many patients of middle age have been embarrassed by their teeth for the whole of their adult life. Many of them say they have had no cosmetic correction until now because they were told as teenagers that 'nothing could be done'. It is worth getting a second (or even a third) opinion if told to grin (how can you?) and bear your unsightly smile.

Disguising unsightly teeth with resin covers

Film actors and actresses used to use, and sometimes still do, a slip of tooth-coloured plastic or porcelain which was fitted over their own, perhaps irregular or stained teeth, during filming. It was not meant to be worn permanently and indeed was stuck into place either by friction or by the use of denture fixative. A newer development which can be considered 'semi-permanent' is the prefabricated resin individual tooth-shaped enamel covers. These are rather similar to the false fingernails which have been in existence for some years. These laminated veneers are of different sizes to match most front teeth and may be trimmed for exact coverage. The patient with malformed (sometimes with too much space between the upper incisors), stained, cracked or fractured teeth, is a good candidate for the application of these veneers. They may be regarded as a 'long-term temporary' improvement, especially for young patients where full crown construction needs to be deferred until the end of their teens. It is also useful for older patients to demonstrate improvements which can be made later with full crown construction, or if the general condition of the patient does not allow him or her to undergo the long sittings necessary for the more permanent restorations.

In use the affected teeth are prepared by cleaning carefully and the enamel is etched by a special weak acid. The enamel becomes porous (a reversible condition) and a resin is applied. This resin is fluid and finds its way into the pores of the enamel and is therefore attached very closely and firmly. The veneers are affixed using a resin paste of the correctly matching colour and bonds to the treated tooth surface after a few minutes. When set, the edges are trimmed with special tiny diamond burs. The patient has to clean the veneers very carefully – too much pressure and rubbing will scratch and eventually wear away some of the surface because these veneers are, of course, softer than enamel.

Patients often forget that the dentist informed them this was a less expensive alternative to crowning, but needed renewing fairly regularly – about two-yearly. The time varies according to the pressure exerted when brushing and the hardness of the bristles. An alternative to these veneers is the use of tooth-coloured resins (similar to the bonding resin used for the veneers) which are applied directly to the acid etched enamel (see above). The colour-matched resin attached to the enamel is built up layer on layer as required. Some resins set by chemical action in about two minutes, others can be painted and moulded and then made to set by the action of a special light emission gun (similar to ultra violet light). The hardened resin, which contains tiny quartz beads to improve the strength, is then shaped and polished. Duration of such totally constructed veneers can be from six months to two years. The difficulty is obtaining a high polish on the surface because the tiny beads tend to leave an irregular surface which later may pick up stain, more in some mouths than others. The patient must therefore be prepared for regular renewal or 'topping up'.

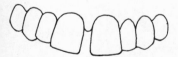 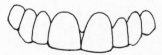

Figure 22. An unsightly gap may be corrected by using modern acid etch composite filling materials as above. This is relatively inexpensive, but requires regular checking.

Protecting your investment

It does not make much sense to spend many hours in the dental chair, pay a considerable fee for an excellent and pleasing cosmetic result and then neglect to take care of your new crowns, bridges and other restorations. Any natural teeth not involved in the restoration work need to be looked after with as much care as ever. It would be foolish to spend time cleaning the new teeth, but allow your own to deteriorate, thus necessitating further expensive work.

Bridgework which has been fixed to the standing teeth cannot be removed for cleaning and, as food and debris may collect underneath it, you must adopt special care methods which the dentist or hygienist will demonstrate to you. With teeth joined together it is impossible to pass dental floss between them from the biting surface, so the floss has to be passed under the bridge teeth using special plastic 'needles'. Floss threaders (Eez-thru, Butler) can be obtained from your local chemist or from the dentist. Other excellent devices are Perio-aid (Butler) which are small brushes like those sold for cleaning cigarette lighters (or like miniature bottle washers). They, too, can be obtained from your chemist or dentist.

If damage to the teeth has been caused by injury to the enamel from regular intake of highly acid lemon juice, or even grapefruit taken as part of a reducing diet, this intake should be stopped or further breakdown will result after cosmetic corrections have been carried out.

17
The Removal of Teeth

In spite of all dentists do in their endeavours to save teeth, there will always be teeth that need to be removed. The milk teeth are usually shed naturally by the process of their roots being resorbed as soon as the successors are ready to erupt through the jaws. Sometimes a milk tooth is not shed and its retention may cause subsequent malalignment of other teeth. Extraction is therefore indicated. Adult teeth which are badly affected by decay and which are not reparable, or those so loosened by periodontal disease, are also scheduled for removal. The orthodontist may recommend the extraction of some quite sound premolar teeth if there does not appear to be sufficient room for them to be retained. Other teeth may become infected and develop cysts and some permanent teeth, principally the third molars (wisdom teeth) and also canines (eye teeth), may be crowded out of the jaws and unable to erupt because of lack of room (impacted teeth). Buried fractured roots may require removal.

Most extractions are simple, but some may be difficult. This will depend on the shape of the roots and the relationship of the tooth to the surrounding structures (other teeth, jawbone – whether covered partially or fully) and on other considerations. The dentist must be properly prepared even for an apparently simple extraction by taking an X-ray of the area and by making a careful visual examination of the involved tooth and surrounding gum. Even the loosest tooth should be X-rayed before extraction because on rare occasions the loosening may be caused by systemic conditions which require investigation by a doctor. The patient's general health and medical history must be checked and a cover of antibiotics given for those needing special care, such as those with heart valve disorders. Other conditions, e.g. diabetes, or the taking of medicines such as anticoagulants, all have a bearing on the procedure which the dentist will adopt before embarking on the extraction. More often than not a local injection is given to anaesthetize the area.

For difficult extractions the dentist may decide on a surgical approach in which the gum is incised and lifted up so that some bone can be removed from around the tooth and the tooth may also be sectioned so that twisted roots of multi-rooted teeth can be removed singly in their most favourable direction of release. The 'flap' of gum is replaced and sutured (stitched) back into position where it heals in a few days. Sutures are usually removed in four days. Having the gum flap lifted to remove a buried root or a difficult tooth is not painful and it is often much better for the dentist to use this method than to continue trying to remove bits of broken tooth with a pair of forceps which he forces into the socket with some pressure. The analogy would be the difference between a difficult forceps delivery of a baby compared to the planned delivery by Caesarian section if problems are envisaged. If complicated surgery is involved, e.g. the removal of four impacted wisdom teeth (see below), or if the patient is very nervous, or prefers it, the operation may be undertaken under general anaesthetic, usually at a hospital where the recovery after the anaesthetic can be monitored. Insurance organizations in most parts of the world usually make provision for payment for the more difficult dental operations such as removal of impactions, cysts, etc.

Wisdom teeth

The wisdom teeth are the last four molar teeth at the back of the mouth, one to each quadrant of the jaws. They erupt into the mouth between the ages of seventeen and twenty-five years approximately. They are the last to grow through and the jaws are sometimes not large enough to accommodate them. The crowding out may take different forms. If you are trying to board an already crowded commuter train and find that it is so full you cannot get in, you may be left standing on the platform; you may alternatively push your way in and find you are half in and out and are blocking the door and thereby causing a good deal of trouble. Finally, you may be able to make your way into the crowded carriage by pushing the other passengers aside. Similarly with wisdom teeth: (1) If they are unable to erupt and are left buried in the bone they may cause very little trouble but should be checked regularly with X-rays because sometimes cysts develop on teeth which have not erupted. (2) If they are half through the gum and are wedged (impacted) so that they can go no further, they may be a source of trouble because bacteria may enter the gum through the opening made by the tooth and cause an infection around the partially erupted wisdom tooth (which is almost impossible to clean). The dentist calls this pericoronitis. (3) Finally, a wisdom tooth may erupt completely, or almost completely, but at the expense of the teeth in front of it.

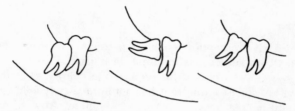

Figure 23. Some types of wisdom tooth positions. The centre one is horizontal and presents some difficulty.

In many people, wisdom teeth come through normally, in a good position and do not cause trouble. Therefore not all wisdom teeth have to be removed. Neither is the removal of wisdom teeth, where necessary, always a problem. Sometimes dentists, quite rightly, and after much consideration, advise the removal of wisdom teeth which have erupted normally into the mouth but, because of lack of room and the impossibility of proper cleaning, are subject to repeated decay or gum inflammation. In this case extraction is usually simple (always checked with radiographs first) and the loss of the teeth is never noticed.

The teeth which generally give trouble and may require surgical intervention are the partly erupted lower impacted wisdom teeth which are obstructed from growing into the mouth because they are striking against the teeth in front, or because the angle of eruption is so unnatural that they cannot completely grow through the bone. The family dentist may be able to tackle this surgery or he may decide to refer the case to an oral surgeon to have the teeth removed. The patient or the surgeon may wish (if all four wisdom teeth are to be removed) to have this done under general anaesthesia.

Other teeth which are sometimes crowded out are the *upper canine teeth*. These are sometimes found by radiographs to be lying in the palate behind the front teeth. If they are causing no trouble, they may, according to the judgement of the dentist, be left in place. Sometimes, if there is a gap in the line of the teeth caused by the absence of canines, the buried teeth may be surgically transplanted to their correct position in the arch and they often remain in a healthy state for many years after their move.

Aftercare

Post-operative discomfort after the extraction of teeth, including wisdom tooth surgery, is minimal these days, but there may be some swelling for two to three days (see below). It is therefore advisable to choose a time which is not immediately followed by an important engagement such as a wedding. Any stitches are removed painlessly on the fourth or fifth day, and by that time any soreness will be diminishing. By the end of ten days healing should be well under way.

Following the more usual tooth removal most extraction sites (sockets) heal without complications. The dentist may hand out a set of instructions together with some gauze and painkilling tablets if required. The instructions usually given to patients are as follows:

1. Bite down on a gauze sponge placed in your mouth for half an hour.

2. Do not rinse for the rest of the day. Tomorrow rinse gently (half a teaspoon of salt to one glass of warm water). Eat soft foods and drink the usual liquids, nothing too hot or too cold.

3. Do not disturb the wound with your tongue or by sucking on the clot.

For discomfort: take two analgesic tablets every four hours. If discomfort persists, call the dentist's office for instructions.

For bleeding: your saliva may be blood-stained for several days. If there is more than a trickle wipe your mouth out with clean gauze or cotton. Place a clean cotton sponge over the bleeding area and bite firmly. Repeat if necessary. A tea bag saturated with warm water is also good.

For swelling: wrap ice chips or cubes in a clean towel and apply to the outside of your face, fifteen minutes on, fifteen minutes off, for three hours. If excessive bleeding, pain, or swelling occurs, call the dentist's office at once.

Avoid doing anything which may disturb the clot in the socket. Therefore rinsing for the first twenty-four hours is *not* advised. Not only will loss of the clot cause continual bleeding but, later on, in a day or two, this may give rise to the very painful condition known as 'dry socket' (see below). It is also advisable, if upper back teeth have been removed, to avoid blowing the nose too vigorously for a few days. This is because sometimes the root tips of these back teeth poke into the nasal sinus (antrum) and vigorous blowing of the nose may force infection through the socket into the sinus. Any pain after the second day is usually due to a dry socket and the dentist should be consulted about this.

'Dry socket'

However excellent the surgery, or however carefully teeth have been removed, some patients get a 'dry socket' which may start about two days after the extraction. Some people are more liable to get dry sockets than others; this may be related to their general health. Dry socket is always due to loss of the blood clot which leads to the unprotected jawbone in the socket becoming inflamed and infected. The condition is usually very painful indeed. There may be a foul smell or a very bad taste. The dentist should be seen as soon as possible. Although the patient has been told not to rinse for twenty-four hours after the extraction one often finds that this advice was ignored and the clot was rinsed away. However, once a dry socket begins, gently rinsing the area to clear food debris out of the socket is important. The dentist will syringe the socket carefully and will usually insert one of the pastes specially formulated to ease the pain and expedite healing. But the victim must be patient because it usually takes about seven to ten days before the bone is sufficiently covered by healing tissue to be protected. If you *do* get a dry socket after extraction do not blame the dentist. It is rarely his fault. It has been said that the clumsy extractor is *less* likely to produce dry sockets, probably because there is much more bleeding after he has finished!

18
The Replacement of Teeth

The main reasons for having teeth replaced are:

Appearance. Not only is the effect of missing teeth in the front of the mouth unsightly but the loss of back teeth will eventually cause a loss of facial height and a falling-in of the cheeks and deepening of lines in the skin, hence a premature ageing of the features. Those who 'don't look their age' at seventy or more have almost certainly retained all their teeth, especially the back ones, to preserve the facial height and therefore muscle and skin tone. The restoration of the tooth-arch shape in width will help to restore facial form.

Biting and chewing. Sometimes the loss of teeth one after another over the years is so gradual that the person does not realize he or she has difficulty masticating food. This may be brought to notice by the occurrence of digestive problems, but there is often a simultaneous gradual change in diet to softer and more easily assimilated food. This has a bad effect on the remaining few teeth, which are liable to be attacked more easily by decay because of the soft diet.

Speech. A gap in the teeth may cause a whistle or other unusual noise during pronunciation. Of course this can also happen with poorly constructed false teeth but a well made tooth replacement will enable normal speech to be restored.

Protection of remaining natural teeth. If missing teeth are not replaced the remaining natural teeth may move out of position into the spaces. If this occurs the upper and lower teeth cannot meet correctly; abnormal forces are then exerted on the teeth which may become loose in their sockets. In the opposite jaw the tooth with nothing to meet tends to grow out of its socket (see

Figure 24). Food will get packed around this tooth and there is the probability of decay and gum disease as a result.

Disturbance of the way in which the teeth meet will cause stress to be placed on the muscles controlling the lower jaw (as already described on page 44).

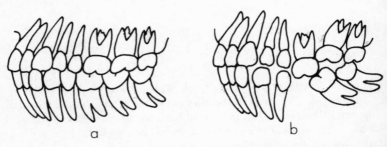

a   b

Figure 24. In (a) the teeth meet normally; (b) shows the possible effects of the non-replacement of one molar tooth.

A well designed partial denture or bridge will help to preserve the strength of the remaining teeth by reducing the load on them and also bracing them if necessary. A poorly designed bridge or denture may put the standing teeth at risk by encouraging food stagnation around them or by irritating the gum surrounding the natural teeth.

Missing teeth can be replaced by the following methods: fixed bridgework; partial removable dentures; overdenture; complete dentures.

Fixed bridgework

This is probably the most desirable method of replacing missing teeth and depends on the presence of healthy, natural teeth on either side of the gap to be 'bridged'. Crowns or inlays are made for these adjoining teeth and the replacements are fixed in with the crowns as one unit, using a special dental cement. Bridges have the advantage that once in position they feel much like the natural teeth and the appearance is good. The disadvantage is high cost and the necessity to 'drill' or otherwise grind the bearing teeth.

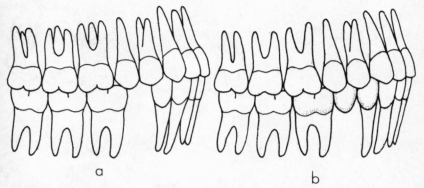

a   b

Figure 25. The missing tooth in (a) is replaced by crowning the teeth on either side of the gap and fixing the bridge tooth to these crowns which are cemented in place (b).

Partial removable dentures

It is often possible, as we have seen, to replace missing teeth by fixed bridgework as long as the natural teeth adjoining are strong enough to bear the extra weight. However, it is not possible to construct fixed bridgework if many teeth are missing or if the

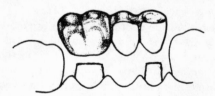

Figure 26. Detail of fixed bridge before insertion.

remaining teeth are too weak to be used as supports. Too long a gap means that the bridge has to span a great distance from one fixed tooth to another. It is like making a bridge across a very wide river with no support in between; it will tend to sag in the middle, and eventually collapse. Thus dentists make partial removable dentures which are supported both by the remaining teeth and by the gum and bone tissues between them. Perhaps the nearest

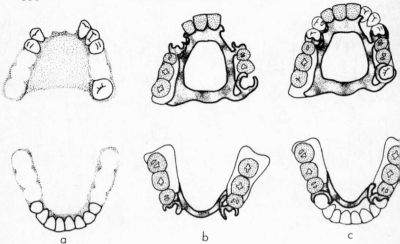

Figure 27. Upper and lower partial metal 'skeleton' (openwork) dentures: (a) the mouth before dentures are fitted, (b) the dentures and (c) the dentures in place attached to the natural teeth. The metal may be chrome-cobalt or gold.

equivalent to our river would be the floating pontoon bridge. Fixing bridgework to weak teeth will eventually cause their loss because of the extra weight they have to bear.

The teeth for removable dental appliances are made of plastic or porcelain which are closely matched in colour and shape to the patient's remaining teeth. They are joined together on a base made of plastic or metal. There are often clasps which attach or grasp the denture to the natural teeth. Sometimes people call these partial dentures 'removable bridges', but dentists usually reserve the term 'bridge' or 'bridgework' for those teeth that are fixed to the natural teeth without a plate.

A partial denture in which the whole of the base is made of plastic may be satisfactory but is generally considered to be of a temporary nature because the plastic has to be wide and cover a large area, because a narrow band of plastic tends to fracture. It is more satisfactory to fit a skeleton (openwork) type of partial denture with as little base as possible, apart from the teeth which are being replaced. This skeleton is cast in metal; the teeth will be in plastic or porcelain, matching the natural ones in colour. The metal casting is usually chrome-cobalt or gold. The high cost of gold today usually indicates a preference for chrome-cobalt. The latter has many advantages: lightness (about half the weight of gold), strength and resistance to corrosion, as well as a lower intrinsic cost.

However, the construction and casting of the metal is probably more difficult than gold, and special laboratories for its processing are usually required. Thus, chrome-cobalt partial dentures are by no means inexpensive if properly constructed.

The advantages of gold are that it is a more versatile metal, and additional parts can be soldered to it later or alterations can be made.

The important consideration in partial dentures is that they should preserve, not destroy the remaining natural teeth. Plastic pieces which irritate the gum immediately surrounding the natural teeth are to be avoided.

There is a belief that clasps which grip the teeth cause decay, but if the teeth are kept clean and free of plaque, and the dentures and clasps are also kept scrupulously clean, the remaining teeth should be safe.

There are many different types of partial dentures and many designs for each individual case. The design and construction of dentures requires skill, and the dentist may decide that the added skills of a specialist, a *prosthodontist,* are required.

Sometimes, when the remaining teeth are loose as a result of periodontal disease, a partial denture may be designed to act as a splint or brace to support these teeth. In this way the loose teeth may have their life prolonged for many years. Your dentist may design the splint himself or he may ask a gum specialist for a design of splint suitable for your condition.

An added luxury and sometimes necessity is the substitution of 'precision attachments' instead of clasps to retain the partial dentures. One or more natural teeth are prepared so that a tiny delicate slotted device is built into them. The denture itself carries a matching attachment which slides exactly into the slot in the natural tooth when the denture is seated in the correct position. This makes a very positive hold for the partial denture. The advantages are that no clasps show from the front of the mouth and the retention is good. Disadvantages are the need to drill and crown the natural teeth receiving the attachment, and the high cost of these attachments, which are nearly always made of gold so that they can be soldered into the crowns and the replacement teeth.

Precision attachments require considerable skill on the part of the dentist and technician and if they are desirable the dentist may ask a specialist to do this work.

Construction of a well made, carefully fitted partial denture may take some time and require many visits to check the accuracy of the casting work. It is not good policy to try to rush the work. Moreover, however quickly a denture is fitted, you will still need time to get used to it. Don't get the idea that in a couple of days you can chew anything or make speeches without any problems at all. These facilities have to be relearned with patience. We do find, however, that if missing *front* teeth are replaced by a partial denture, almost everyone gets on well very quickly. This is because no one wants to go around with gaps in the front and so just has to make the effort, which is proof enough of how important is application and learning. The dentist can help, but in the long run the patient has to do the job himself. Appearance is perhaps not so important when back teeth only are fitted, and often if the wearer gets some slight discomfort he or she gives up and takes the denture out and puts it in the drawer or in a pocket. It would almost be a good idea if dentists always removed just one front tooth with these back teeth so the patient would be made to wear the denture; and then they are certain to have a co-operative patient who will get on very quickly and be able to wear back teeth; but of course, this is not an ethical consideration.

The new denture, however well made, is a 'foreign body' in the mouth. The tongue trips up on it and, even if small and delicate, it still feels bulky to the cheeks and tongue, and there may be difficulty in pronouncing and articulating certain words. There is excessive salivation with probable dribbling, because the presence of something strange in the mouth makes the saliva glands believe it is food and so there is an excessive flow. This will correct itself as the mouth adapts to the denture. Adaptation is accomplished by wearing the appliance and using it, not by putting it in a drawer. If, after continuous practice, there is still discomfort or problems in eating or speaking, tell your dentist; but there should be no attempt to carry out do-it-yourself dentistry on the denture.

It is foolhardy to try to alter or bend the clasps or any part of the denture. The denture may be damaged and, more important, there may be damage to the supporting teeth. If there are any problems, they should be explained to the dentist, and he will make any necessary adjustments without charge for a reasonable time after the fitting has been made.

Inserting and removing partial dentures should be practised while with the dentist at the time they are fitted. At first you may find difficulty putting them in and taking them out, but once you have done it, every repetition becomes easier. Never panic while you are removing the dentures and don't tug at them. Nothing will be accomplished except possibly damage to the teeth and the dentures. Learn to remove and replace them slowly and calmly, always repeating to yourself that if you've done it once, you can do it again.

One of the main complaints received by the dentist when partial dentures have been worn for a few days is that food gets trapped round the metalwork and they need to be cleaned after every meal. After a week or two these complaints cease, although the dentist has made no alteration to the dentures. What has happened is that in this short time the tongue has learned to carry out the normal cleansing action around the new dentures.

It is foolish to spend time cleaning your dentures (for the correct method see Complete dentures below) while neglecting your natural teeth. These must be scrupulously brushed and cleaned more carefully than ever because of the dangers of food trapping which has been mentioned above.

The mouth itself changes periodically, so that regular check-ups by the dentist are necessary. Alterations to the bases of the dentures may be indicated to compensate for any shrinkage that might have occurred.

The overdenture

This is a fairly new version of an old technique and its use is rapidly changing the whole concept of denture making, possibly reducing to insignificant numbers the incidence of extractions of all the teeth. Those dentists who have taken to making overdentures now save the roots of many of the teeth they previously would have extracted.

The overdenture is in effect a complete denture (or often a conventional partial denture, too); it is supported not only by the gums but also by the remaining natural teeth which are completely covered over by the denture. The natural teeth, which have been grossly damaged or weakened by gum disease, are shortened or altered in shape to stumps which allow the denture to fit snugly over them. Retaining the teeth prevents the bone shrinkage which would have taken place had the roots been extracted, and the stumps help retention of the denture which is much better than with the conventional complete denture. Moreover, it is often possible, after further treatment of one or more of the stumps, to insert what is rather like a snap-fastener attachment in the root and the denture. Thus very weak remaining teeth which normally would not be capable of supporting a partial denture can be made to serve a useful purpose.

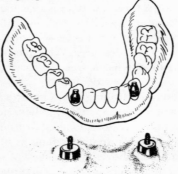

Figure 28. Overdenture. This has attachments built into it which snap on to corresponding members inserted into roots remaining in the jaw. The retention is usually excellent. (*Courtesy of Dr H.W. Preiskel*)

The dentist may reduce the natural teeth by a small amount, as if constructing a crown, or by a greater amount down to a level with the gums. In the latter case it will be necessary to remove the pulp from the remaining part of the tooth root.

The prospective full-denture patient should therefore ask the dentist about the possibilities of overdentures. There is nothing to lose because overdentures cannot do harm and usually do a great deal of good. The worst that could happen in the event of the fracture or decay of the retained roots is that complete dentures could be finally constructed. By that time the patient will be used to the feel and idea of the denture which would then give little trouble.

Complete or full dentures

When all the teeth have been lost the replacement is called a complete or full denture. It is possible to have a complete denture in one jaw and natural teeth in the opposite jaw; however, a 'set' of full dentures, both upper and lower, may be necessary. The shape of the upper denture is different from the lower because it is made to cover the hard palate behind the front teeth, while the space between the teeth on the lower jaw is occupied by the tongue and important structures in the floor of the mouth (under the tongue), so the denture must be kept away from this region (see Figure 30).

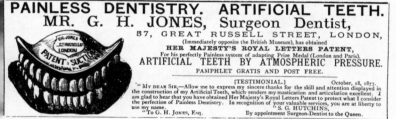

Figure 29. Newspaper advertisement for dentures, *c.* 1870. (*Mary Evans Picture Library*)

Because it is broader, and covers a wider area, the upper denture is more stable and more comfortable. It does not fall downwards because there is a great deal of adhesion resulting from the wide area of coverage. A similar sort of adhesion occurs between two wet flat sheets of glass. They are very difficult to pull apart. The bond between the two faces is great because the film of water between them exerts enormous surface tension and because the atmospheric pressure holds the two sheets together. The bigger the sheet, the more adhesion there is, and the same is true of an upper denture. Therefore the dentist tries to extend the upper denture over as wide an area as possible, although the wearer might think it better to have it as small as possible!

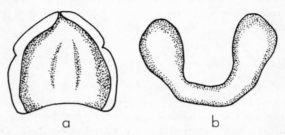

Figure 30. The reverse side (the fitting surface) of (a) an upper and (b) a lower denture showing the difference in tissue coverage.

In the pre-World War II days of 'blood and vulcanite', as dentistry was then called, the British dentist gained a world-wide reputation as someone who preferred to extract all the teeth and make dentures. This was largely true and the emphasis in most dental schools throughout the world was on the making of false teeth. As students we spent two years of our four-year course working in the dental laboratory learning how to make different forms of tooth replacement. Pre-World War II dentures were made of vulcanized rubber instead of the very natural-looking plastic of today. The colour and taste of the vulcanite were poor, and processing and repair were complicated. The teeth were porcelain with little metal pins in the backs of them to attach them to the vulcanite. These porcelain teeth tended to click when they came together. Today's plastic teeth are 'silent' and are attached to the plastic base of the denture by a chemical bond.

Artificial teeth *can* be made so perfectly today that it would be difficult or impossible for most people to distinguish them from natural teeth, but this cannot be done for everyone.

Making a set of false teeth calls for a great deal of skill, care, patience, tact, and scientific knowledge, allied to an artistic sense. To this must be added the ability to deal with the understandable mental trauma associated with the loss of teeth. Dentures are not something you buy like a piece of furniture or even a car. The dentures have to satisfy the following requirements:

1. They must fit the jaws *exactly*.

2. There must be no pain or discomfort after the breaking-in period.

3. They must function *many* times every day, enabling satisfactory biting, chewing and swallowing, year after year.

4. Speech must not be affected.

5. They must stay in place without moving.

6. The appearance must be natural, relative to the age of the wearer, in shape, arrangement and the colour of the teeth.

7. Each set must be specially made for each person.

8. They must please the patient.

Can you think of another man-made item that has to satisfy so many exacting requirements? A suit of clothes has to 'fit' but there is considerable tolerance about the fit. As long as we like its appearance and it does not fall apart after a few weeks, we are happy to go on wearing the suit for several years (according to fashion), and yet an 'off the peg' suit from the multiple store tailors costs a great deal more than the dentist is paid for the provision of dentures under many fixed insurance fee schedules, e.g. the National Health Service.

The making of the denture

No one wants to go around without front teeth, even for a short while, so the dentist will arrange to make and insert what is called an *immediate denture* (or dentures). The immediate dentures are constructed in the following stages:

1. Radiographs should be available of all the remaining teeth and also of areas where teeth appear to be missing, in case there are buried roots which might give trouble later.

2. Impressions of both jaws are taken for the construction of study models and to record the manner in which the jaws meet.

3. The back teeth behind the canine teeth are removed together with buried roots, if any.

4. After a suitable healing interval of a few weeks (perhaps four to six) new impressions are taken in special impression trays which were made from the original models of the mouth.

5. A registration is made in the mouth, using special wax blocks

on fitting plates, of the way in which the upper and lower jaws contact each other. This is checked in the laboratory with the original models. The required shape, size and colour of the teeth is noted.

6. The dental technician sets up the 'try-in' stage in which the teeth are set in wax on moulded bases. The front teeth are missing from these trial plates because the natural teeth are still present in the mouth. However, if the arrangement and shade are acceptable to the patient and the occlusion (meeting of the jaws) is satisfactory, the trial plates are returned to the technician for finishing in acrylic material. Note that in the trial stage the back teeth only will appear in the finished set. The dentures will not fit firmly until they have been moulded in hard plastic.

7. The technician removes the remaining front teeth from the plaster model and substitutes the new teeth, making an improved cosmetic appearance if necessary. The dentures are then processed so that the wax and bases are replaced by plastic.

When the dentist decides that the dentures are ready for insertion, the gums are numbed by a local injection (the patient may decide to have the remaining teeth out while under general anaesthetic but this is not necessary from a technical point of view in most cases). The teeth are extracted and the gums are still numb when the new denture or dentures are inserted. The dentist will make any adjustments necessary to ensure that the dentures are comfortable and that they meet each other exactly. He will not dismiss the patient until he thinks the appearance and fit are good.

It is better if the upper denture has artificial gum in the front. Although the lip may feel pushed out a little with the false gum, it improves the retention of the denture and protects the bone underneath. It was the custom previously to allow the tips of the false teeth to protrude into the extraction sockets and although this may have seemed attractive·to the patient, since the teeth appeared to come out of the gum, it had a bad effect on the jaws, preventing healing and distorting the gum. So try to put up with false gum in front. It also helps in the later relining of the denture when it becomes necessary because of the shrinkage of the jaw after extraction.

When the dentures are in place for the first time, the patient is often disappointed. There seems to be such a mouthful. There are two possible side-effects (which with ninety-five per cent of patients are just temporary). These are, first, extra saliva in the mouth and, second, a tendency to gag and retch.

The cause of excess saliva is described on page 152.

The gagging or retching, though rare, can be distressing. Some people also experience nausea when the impressions are taken. They have a fear of anything tickling the back of the throat (the doctor examining the throat with a spatula can be torture to them). It is interesting that more than fifty per cent of these gaggers are non-swimmers – they have a horror of water at the back of their throats. Usually the sufferer asks the dentist to cut the back of the artificial palate shorter. This does little to help, and merely makes the denture looser. Many of these gagging problems are caused not by a sensitive palate, but by the denture tickling the back of the tongue. However, in nearly all cases the gag reflex disappears if the denture is worn for a few days. If the trouble persists, the matter must be discussed with the dentist. As much of the problem is in the patient's mind rather than his mouth, some dentists have occasionally tried hypnosis with success.

The immediate insertion denture should be kept in place for at least twenty-four hours after the extractions and fitting. This will keep the blood clot in the sockets and prevent bleeding. If there is discomfort two analgesic tablets four-hourly for the first day will be helpful. After twenty-four hours the denture may be removed *carefully,* the mouth rinsed and the denture scrubbed and re-inserted. But again, very carefully! The wearer should try to manipulate the denture around the bumps where the canine teeth were. These prominences in the jaws are below the nostrils on both sides, and they are the most common places for soreness after the fitting of the immediate dentures. The dentist may give some ointment to put on the denture at these spots (it is better and easier to put the ointment on the denture rather than to try to get it onto the slippery gum surface). There are a number of special ointments containing soothing substances plus a slight surface anaesthetic called 'benzocain'. A few of them are obtainable directly from your chemist.

It is usually recommended that the new teeth are worn day and night for the first week or two to get used to them. Before going to bed the dentures should be removed, carefully rinsed, and put back. After the first couple of weeks the dentures should be removed at night because the mouth tissues will be relieved of pressure for a few hours. Moreover during the night stagnation takes place under the dentures allowing bacteria to multiply which may lead to a bad taste or even bad breath. However, these recommendations must be overruled by common sense. Few wives or husbands today wish to confront their bedmate with grinning gums, even at night. The decision must be made by the patient in such cases.

Shrinkage and relining

There may be so much shrinkage after a few weeks that the denture, which at first was tight and difficult to get in and out without soreness, is now quite loose. As a temporary measure the wetted inside surface can be sprinkled with some denture fixative powder. The dentist prefers to wait as long as possible before relining the denture, because if it is done too early there will be more shrinkage and a further need for relining. A first reline can be done in cold plastic material, usually while the patient waits. The soft plastic material (which has a burning sensation in the mouth) is placed in the denture and put into the mouth, moulding a new fitting surface which gets hard in a few minutes. The new surface is trimmed and polished and will serve until there is further shrinkage.

However, the upper denture will settle up higher as shrinkage takes place, and eventually it may not be possible to see the teeth very easily, even while smiling. Sometimes the dentist may make the front teeth of the immediate denture slightly longer at the time of insertion to compensate for this shrinkage so that there will still be a good-looking smile. But patients sometimes ask for these teeth to be shortened from the start and in spite of explanations they insist on the shortening. In a few weeks they complain of the 'disappearing teeth'!

The second set

The teeth start to recede under the level of the lip so gradually that the patient gets used to the appearance. Later, when the dentist comes to make the second set the patient may object to his bringing the line of the teeth back to their original level. When the gums have had their major shrinkage and the dentist feels that the patient is ready for the 'main set' (any time from six months to a year after the last extraction) he will take impressions, but this time the teeth will be seen at the wax stage for approval before they are finished.

At this trial stage the position of the teeth can be adjusted or the shade changed. The plate is not yet in hard moulded plastic but in a form of wax; it will not therefore feel snug and tight in the mouth.

The dentist is interested in two things at this stage: how the teeth look in the mouth and how well the teeth in the upper jaw mesh with the lowers as they close together. If everything is agreeable to him and to the patient the wax dentures will be returned to the laboratory for processing on to the completed bases. This try-in stage is crucial. It is at this point that opinions must be expressed because by the next stage it will be too late for much change. It is better to ask the dentist for one more try a few days later than to allow dentures to be finished when you don't have absolute confidence in their appearance.

Living with your dentures

On average a full set of dentures can exert only about one-tenth of the force of natural teeth. Therefore even the best dentures will be a disappointment if too much is expected. The wearer has to learn to adapt to the differences in biting and chewing ability and will benefit if a few 'tricks' or rules are observed. Because of its shape the lower denture is less stable than the upper and so more discomfort is initially felt in the lower. Some commercial firms who market denture fixatives and cleansers issue helpful booklets with advice about wear and care of dentures. These booklets can often be picked up from your dentist.

Remember, learning to wear a denture takes time, so do not

listen to friends who tell you how easy it was for them. They are probably bragging or their memories are poor (or they were just *lucky*). Follow your dentist's advice and don't become discouraged. A complete lower denture takes longer to master than a complete upper. (The tongue may feel restricted, but don't worry, it will soon become accustomed to its new position.)

Eat carefully and slowly. The longer you take over a meal the quicker you will master your dentures.

Cut all food into small portions at first so that you don't have to take large bites. *You will find chewing much easier if you do not chew on one side only* but place small portions of food on both sides at the same time. This is not *natural* chewing but it will balance your dentures and if you learn this, you will have largely mastered chewing. Press down with your finger on the teeth of your lower denture at the back on one side. It will tend to lift up on the other side, which shows how important it is to balance food on both sides. It is probably easier at the start to eat crisp foods like toast rather than sticky foods like soft bread.

Any pressure on the dentures *backwards* into your mouth tends to make the dentures hold more firmly, but a forward pull will tend to dislodge any dentures – try putting your finger behind the front teeth of the bottom set and pulling forward – your teeth will flick out! But now put the same finger on top and slightly on the front of your lower teeth and press downwards and backwards. Your teeth should be firm and stable. From this you can learn how to bite apples and crusts. Normally the natural teeth bite through an apple which is pulled away from the mouth at the same time in a tearing motion. This would of course pull the teeth *forward* with it. So in biting through an apple push it in towards your mouth until your teeth have actually separated the piece. Then you can remove the rest of the apple. Practise this.

Speech may be difficult to begin with, but dentures have never affected the singing of opera stars like Caruso, so when the lips and the tongue have got used to their new neighbours they will adapt to speaking clearly. Practise reading aloud in front of a mirror and note the tongue positions. Dentures are kept in place by a combined effort of your cheeks, lips and tongue. Once these accept the dentures and function with them you have won the battle. The dentist will help you if you have soreness and will deal with other problems that arise but *you* are the only one who can make the effort necessary to win this battle, which need only take a few days with luck and persistence.

Cleaning your dentures

Plaque and tartar form on your denture just as they do on natural teeth. Plastic is slightly absorbent so that if dentures are not cleaned regularly they can become smelly or taste poorly. Strict cleaning preferably after every meal with a *soft* brush and some good denture paste is necessary. Remember that dentures can be broken, so clean them over a bowl of cold water and if the denture slips it will not hit the hard basin; its fall will be broken by the water.

If you grip the horseshoe-shaped lower denture in the palm of the hand it can fracture (this is a common cause of fractured lowers) so hold it gently while brushing.

If the denture is out of the mouth for any length of time it should be kept moist either in water or a cleaning solution. Never keep dentures wrapped in a tissue, e.g. Kleenex; it's liable to be thrown away! Never place dentures in *hot* water – plastic is liable to warp.

There are many denture cleaners in the stores. The one that suits your dentures is found by trial. But basically there are three convenient types:

Alkaline peroxides. These are powder or tablets which are dissolved in water. The dentures are placed in the solution to soak overnight. There is an oxygen liberating agent in these cleaners and a detergent. They are effective and can cause little harm to the dentures. Examples are Steradent, Dentural, Librox, Oxydent.

Acid cleansers (five per cent hydrochloric acid). These are applied with a sponge or a brush and after a short while the fluid is washed off. They are quite effective but if there is a partial denture with metal clasps, corrosion could take place. Examples are Denclen, Densol, Dentyr Bleach.

Abrasives. These are like toothpastes and are brushed on the denture. They should be used with care because the surface of the teeth can be damaged by abrasion. Examples are Dentucreme, Lustre Dent, Dentrfresh.

Information and advice for denture wearers

1. I have pointed out the amount of time and skill needed to fit complete dentures. Therefore, on the whole you get what you pay for.

2. Pain under new dentures often passes off after a few days. If it persists the dentist can adjust the denture in the painful region. Often he will not touch the part that covers the gum, but will grind the artificial tooth over the spot because his tests may show that here the upper and lower teeth are contacting each other before the others, so transmitting pain to the gum underneath.

Persistent pain after adjustments may be caused in the lower jaw if there has been so much shrinkage of the bone that a large nerve which crosses the jaw is reached by the shrinkage, allowing the denture to press on it. The dentist may fit a special soft cushion lining into the denture. In rare cases there may be a need for surgery, in which case a new channel is made in the bone to enclose the nerve.

Pain caused under old dentures indicates that they no longer fit, and the edges may ulcerate parts of the mouth. Once the dentures have been made to fit, or the edges of the dentures are cleared away from the painful ulcerated area, there should be a careful check to ensure that healing of the ulcer has taken place. Persistent ulcerations after alterations to the denture should be investigated by the dentist or an expert in oral medicine.

3. Having teeth out and fitting dentures is not the end of your dental troubles. It is just a change. If you want to maintain a youthful appearance the dentures must be renewed and re-constructed at regular intervals. One-third of the adult population in the UK wear dentures, with disproportionately large numbers of edentulous (i.e. those with no natural teeth) people living in the north of England and Scotland. Because so many people in the north wear full dentures, and because they have been wearing the same dentures for too long, one notices the shrunken faces of masses of people over the age of forty in that area.

4. A common cause of denture fracture is shrinkage of the gums underneath. The denture does not sit evenly in the mouth and the constant flexing of the plastic as it wobbles during mastication will eventually cause a fracture.

Fractures of complete *upper* dentures occur most frequently when the lower natural teeth are still in place. The teeth in the lower jaw, which is the moveable one, smack up against the weaker static set and eventually split the upper denture. This may be a source of dispute between dentist and patient because the latter does not understand why his or her denture should fracture so often while friends and neighbours (who may have full sets of upper and lower artificial teeth) do not have such trouble. Of course the brutal answer would be 'have all your bottom teeth out and that will solve your problems'.

Sometimes, in order to avoid the fracture of the plastic palate, it is replaced by a thin cast metal one. Even this does not always prevent denture fracture but it is worth trying, although the metal adds considerably to the cost.

5. Beware of the denturist – the unqualified mechanic who says he will make you a set of teeth 'on the cheap'. Some denturists might be able to, but most can't. A sore gum under an old denture is usually caused by an ill-fitting denture but it *could* be a malignancy. The dentist must examine all patients carefully. His early spotting of trouble could save a life. So until denturists are licensed, and work with dentists, one should keep away from them.

6. A much stronger objection applies to denture repair shops where 'quick repairs' to broken dentures are promised. Very often these operators try to get the victim to have a reline or remodel or 'duplicate' dentures or even new dentures illegally. Although some of these shops are genuine, many of them are 'cowboys'. 'Cowboy' dental repair shops reap their harvest when someone breaks a denture just before going to a wedding or an important engagement at the weekend. Therefore, always have a spare denture made by your dentist. It has a great number of uses, not only in times of breakage but also when the worn dentures need relining.

7. If you feel your dentures are becoming loose in your mouth, see the dentist as soon as possible. Do not waste time and money on relining kits which the chemist may stock. They may damage not only the dentures but the tissues of the mouth as well. If they were any good your dentist would be using them. (See also Chapter 6 , Home Remedies.)

8. One day you will realize suddenly that you have forgotten that you wear dentures. That is when you will have succeeded. All you will require after that is a regular check-up to see that everything is going well.

If you have not cleaned your dentures effectively they will get encrusted with tartar like the fur in a kettle. If the crust forms *inside* the denture where it should touch the gum your denture does not fit and needs a reline. If your denture is all plastic, and contains no metal, you can try removing the hard crust on it by immersing it in warm *white* vinegar (acetic acid) for about half an hour. Then brush off the softened tartar and wash the dentures carefully under running water. If your denture stains easily it may mean that you're brushing them too fiercely, either with a hard brush or an abrasive paste, and have removed the polished surface, enabling the stain to be picked up easily. See the dentist who may be kind enough to get your dentures repolished by his technician.

Implant dentures

Some people who have not succeeded in overcoming denture problems ask whether they can be fitted with implant dentures. But few dentists provide implant dentures and the costs are usually very high. Surgery is carried out on the jaws and a metal framework is buried under the gums with vertical rods projecting through the gums to bear a denture sitting on these rods. This is called a *sub-periosteal implant*. Dental implants differ from all other implants (such as hip replacements) in that the others are *closed* in the body while dental implants provide direct contact between the mouth (and its bacteria) and the jawbone underneath. While some dental implants have succeeded for a reasonable time, many dentists do not consider that they are yet an acceptable risk. The penalty of failure of the implant may be considerable destruction of the jawbone around the metalwork of the implant.

The *endosseous implant* is usually made up of single implants which are set *into* the bone, instead of the previously mentioned implant which sits *on* the bone. They may be in the form of blades which are embedded in the jawbones through the gum, and have studs or other projections through the gum in order to take a crown or part of a fixed bridge or denture. The same arguments apply to these as to the sub-periosteal implant.

I personally would not undergo an implant operation. However, great strides are being made and future developments may mean that implants will become a generally recognized part of restorative dentistry.

Insuring against accident or loss

Much dental treatment is very expensive and is becoming even more expensive with the enormous increases in the cost of essential materials such as gold and silver.

People lose their dentures and accidents occur in which expensive dental restorations are fractured and have to be remade. Therefore consideration should be given to insuring such dentistry and there are a number of companies who will take on the risk. You will not be able to insure against loss caused by further dental decay or deterioration or loss of teeth, e.g. due to gum disease, which hold the insured appliance in place.

Preferentially the work should be covered as soon as it is completed, or inserted, but usually the insurers will accept work up to two years old provided the dentist certifies the age of the work and that it is in 'perfect condition' (very difficult to define!) at the time of proposal.

One of the ways of avoiding insurance premiums is to take care that accidents do not happen. Although some accidents are inevitable, occasionally they are the result of carelessness. One of the most frequent cases reported to us is the loss of dentures, especially small partial dentures of chrome-cobalt or gold which may take up little space, but are inevitably expensive. The paper tissue (or Kleenex) is the real danger. *Never* wrap anything of value in paper tissues. They are often rolled up and thrown away, especially in hotels by enthusiastic chamber maids. Bridgework, which may be fixed in your mouth so that you cannot lose it, may nevertheless be damaged by accident from a blow. Insurance is wise in this instance. Your dentist will advise you. If you have an *all risks* Home Insurance you may find that your dental appliances can be covered, or anyway you can extend cover for an additional sum. It may be a lot cheaper than any of the 'special dental insurances' offered today.

19
Going Abroad

It is remarkable how many travellers encounter problems that necessitate urgent medical or dental attention while they are abroad. Many of the problems occur without warning symptoms. Warning symptoms might have been there but were of a minor nature and were ignored. I remember having my *first* attack of gout while in Rome and my wife had her *first* attack of a particularly nasty stomach disorder at the same time. Careful diagnosis on return revealed that in both cases the underlying causes had been present for some time but the sudden change in diet, combined in my case with more walking than I had been used to, precipitated the attacks.

A thorough medical check-up would have revealed my problem before leaving and prophylactic tablets could have prevented the attack. However, in my wife's case, the most careful pre-vacation examination would not have revealed her problem, which was a rare one.

If we interpret this in terms of dental care, a thorough dental examination and correction of any teeth likely to give trouble while you're away is obviously the sensible course to adopt. Those who have a regular dental check-up and have been passed as dentally fit in the last few months should be free of dental problems. If you have had no dental attention for an extensive period (over twelve months) a booking should be made with your family dentist *well before* the date of your vacation. In view of the problems of booking appointments and in case some extensive work requires to be done it is wise to book about two months before your departure.

However, even with careful dental attention at home it is still possible for problems to arise abroad, many of them of an accidental nature. A tooth can fracture on a hard piece of bone, or a denture can break. Indulging in games or sports may cause accidental damage. Note that fracture of teeth in youngsters occurs in swimming pools with surprising frequency.

Some of these problems *can* be avoided by extra care, and denture wearers should always have a spare set with them. Most people, even the very wealthy, have an odd sense of priority. Many of them would not dream of having a spare set of teeth ('the dentist is trying to put one over on me') even though they have an extra colour TV in the bedroom and certainly own more than one suit or dress.

Good care of the mouth before going abroad should involve the following: all decayed cavities should be cleaned out (excavated) and filled with a long-lasting sedative temporary dressing, if completion is not possible in the time available. Your teeth should be cleaned very thoroughly so that there is no inflammation around the gums. The dentist or hygienist may need two or three visits to accomplish this satisfactorily. You are then less likely to contract a gum infection.

One problem that can arise suddenly in teenagers is the infected wisdom tooth. It may be partly erupted with a flap of gum covering part of it. Bacteria breed under this flap at the back of the mouth and may flare up, causing a severe infection and swelling. A survey of the dental state of the athletic teams competing in the Olympic Games in Mexico indicated that infected wisdom teeth were responsible for a great deal of trouble and, in one instance, a world record holder was unable to compete because of a grossly infected jaw. It may seem drastic, but if your dentist considers that wisdom teeth may give trouble they should be dealt with, often by extraction, or he may prescribe special mouthwashes or antibiotics which can be taken with you as a safety measure.

Dental attention in a foreign country is needed either in emergency by the temporary visitor or as routine treatment by prospective residents.

The dental attention required by the temporary visitor is likely to be for the relief of pain. There are of course unfortunate occurrences, including motor or skiing accidents, which may call for extensive immediate treatment, but this would be a hospital matter and fractured jaws, for example, would probably be dealt with in conjunction with any other injuries.

The following are the main points of concern in obtaining emergency treatment: finding a dentist; getting an early appointment; communicating; limiting the work to the area of immediate concern; paying the bill.

Finding a dentist in one's own country is difficult enough, especially when one needs immediate or early attention for a toothache. Dentists' appointments are carefully planned and emergency calls for the relief of pain upset the schedule. But many dentists do mark off a period each day for unscheduled visits and a telephone call in an emergency may well be successful.

First you have to find your dentist. If you are staying in a hotel the most obvious and frequently used method is to ask the head porter. Certainly in this country most hotels keep a list of local doctors and dentists. The dentist contacted is likely to be expensive but because of his desire to oblige the hotel he will probably find you an appointment. In the UK doctors and dentists would be guilty of unprofessional conduct if they entered into any sort of arrangement with hotels and other organizations for the referral of patients, but measures adopted in other countries may differ. If you have friends or business acquaintances nearby they may be of assistance in obtaining an appointment. They would almost certainly know of a practitioner and might have enough personal 'pull' to obtain an early appointment. Other sources of help would be the local Consulate or Embassy which may carry a medical or dental list. The advantage here would be that the list often contains the names of English-speaking and/or UK- or USA-trained dentists.

If there are going to be language problems make sure that you take with you a good modern phrase-book. Today's phrase-books are very simple to use and cover almost any situation that may arise. One of the best series is published by Berlitz in many languages. At the end of this chapter is a sample 'starter' kit of simple phrases in the basic languages of countries where the natives may not (and sometimes today *will not*) speak English. Languages like Dutch, Swedish, Danish have not been included because so many of the dentists in those countries speak English.

If you fail to find a dentist who will give you treatment ask for the address and telephone number of the university hospital. It probably has a dental department or dental school attached.

Once you have found your dentist and made the appointment, be sure you know how to get to his premises and how far away they are. A taxi ride from one side of Paris to the other could be very expensive, so if you are in a large town try to choose someone who is fairly near in case you have to return for further visits. The hall porter's or receptionist's lists are particularly useful in this respect because they are likely to recommend people in the near vicinity.

At your appointment be sure to tell the dentist if you have any medical condition which requires special care such as diabetes, heart condition, etc. (if you are a 'bleeder' you should preferably attend a hospital), and let him know whether you have any allergies or are taking any pills or medicines.

Here again a phrase-book such as the Berlitz is invaluable because it lists all these conditions in the medical section and all you need do is point to the relevant names in the book or, better still, copy them out in advance. Try to make sure that you have the minimum work done sufficient to remove your pain or restore your appearance (e.g. refixing a crown on a front tooth). If you are returning home in a few days even an abscessed tooth may respond to antibiotics until you can see your own dentist. However, this is a matter for the judgement of the dentist you are seeing and your feelings about his advice. You should not allow him to embark on a series of fillings or complicated expensive restorations such as crowns unless you are convinced of the necessity for their being done before you return home.

With regard to a crown in the front of the mouth which comes loose, if this is on a metal post which inserts into the root, the dentist should make sure that the crown has not loosened because of a split in your root. If he does not notice this and cements the crown back into the split root you will almost certainly suffer severe pain and possibly an abscess eventually. In such an event make sure that the dentist takes a radiograph.

You should always organize cover for medical expenses abroad as part of your travel arrangements. The cover should be for as large an amount as you can afford. Medical and dental expenses are usually very high for tourists in every country you are likely to visit. It is worth enquiring whether emergency dental charges will be covered.

If you are a prospective resident or long-stay visitor abroad you have to choose between finding a dentist in the country where you are staying and arranging routine treatment and check-ups on return trips home. This must be a personal decision.

If you decide to look for a dentist in your new habitat the same problems will apply as at home, and almost the same methods of introduction are needed. If you are replacing an employee or executive he might be able to refer you to the dentist who looked after him.

In deciding whether to have regular treatment abroad or to return home you must consider the general reputation of the dentistry in the country in which you are living. I intended to give here a table of 'good' and 'bad' dental countries, but I have been told it might precipitate an international incident! However, it can be said that, *if you can get an appointment,* you should be reasonably confident of finding a good dentist in the Netherlands, Germany, the Scandinavian countries, Switzerland, Austria, France, Australia, New Zealand, Canada, Mexico, USA, South Africa and many other countries.

There are variable standards in all countries and in those countries which have not been mentioned superb dentists exist but they may not be thick on the ground and often the standards of dental education do not conform with ours.

In any country a good tip is to look for a dentist who has had a post-graduate degree at a university dental school in the USA, Canada, the UK or Australia.

Your dentist at home may be able to advise you about an acceptable dentist in your new country. There are several useful international lists.

Some Useful Phrases

ENGLISH	FRENCH	GERMAN	SPANISH	ITALIAN
Can you speak English?	Parlez-vous anglais?	Sprechen Sie Englisch?	¿Habla usted inglés?	Parla inglese?
I have a toothache.	J'ai mal aux dents.	Ich habe Zahnschmerzen	Tengo dolor de muelas.	Ho mal di denti.
Can you recommend a good dentist?	Pouvez-vous me recommànder un bon dentiste?	Können Sie einen guten Zahnarzt empfehlen?	¿Puede recomendarme un buen dentista?	Puo consigliarmi un buon dentista?
Can I make an appointment to see Dr...?	Puis-je prendre un rendez-vous avec le docteur?	Kann ich einen Termin bei Herrn Dr... ausmachen?	¿Puedo pedir cita para ver al doctor...?	Desidero un appuntamento con il dottore.
Can't you make it earlier?	Ne pourriez-vous pas me prendre plus tôt?	Können Sie das nicht früher machen?	¿No sería posible antes?	Non è possibile prima?
I have lost a filling.	J'ai perdu un plombage.	Ich habe eine Füllung verloren.	Me he perdido un empasto	L'otturazione si è staccata
This tooth hurts.	Cette dent me fait mal.	Dieser Zahn schmerzt.	Me duele este diente.	Mi fa male questo dente.

At the top, bottom, front, back.	En haut, en bas, devant, derrière.	Oben, unten, vorne, hinten.	Arriba, abajo, delante, detrás.	In alto, in basso, davanti, dietro.
Can you fix it temporarily?	Pouvez-vous faire un traitement provisoire?	Können Sie ihn provisorisch behandeln?	¿Puede usted arreglarlo temporalmente?	Puo curarlo provvisoriamente?
The gum is sore.	La gencive est douloureuse.	Das Zahnfleisch ist wund.	Las encías están inflamadas.	La gengiva è infiammata.
I've broken my denture.	J'ai cassé mon dentier.	Mein Gebiss ist zerbrochen.	Se me ha roto la dentadura.	Ho rotto mia dentiera.
When will it be ready?	Quand sera-t-il prêt?	Wann ist es fertig?	¿Cuando estará hecha?	Quando sara pronta?
How much do I owe you?	Combien vous dois-je?	Wieviel schulde ich Ihnen?	¿Cuanto le debo?	Quanto le devo?

20
Some Recent Developments and Trends

Research, both in relation to the actual treatment of patients and to the improvement in dental materials and equipment has made enormous progress in the last few years. These developments are often brought into use quite quickly and thus anyone writing about today's dentistry soon finds that early revision has to be made.

Some of the developments which have currently been adopted in practice are discussed below. Other developments may not yet be readily available in the average practice.

Fillings

Silver amalgam, used in back teeth (see page 117) has a number of admirable qualities. When carefully inserted into the tooth cavity it makes a fine restoration which can be carved and polished and is reasonably inexpensive – the main disadvantages are the appearance and the tendency for the material to be brittle in thin sections. Silver amalgam, even with the development of tooth-coloured posterior filling materials, must still be considered as the best general-purpose filling of choice. The wear properties of amalgam fillings have been improved by changes in the metallic chemistry with a considerable increase in the amount of copper in the filling powder. Looking into the future there may be some doubt as to the continued use of these fillings because they depend on mercury for mixing into a soft mass for ease of insertion into the tooth cavity. The reserves of mercury are limited, and as it is a toxic material there is some concern that, although patients are free from danger, some dental staff may occasionally be exposed to hazard from careless handling.

Tooth-coloured fillings

(Composite fillings see page 119)

These materials are being improved almost daily and specially developed fillings which look good are being used by some dentists in the molar teeth. Many big industrial companies such as ICI, 3M, etc, are producing such fillings and the long-term testing in the dental schools has been quite favourable. One of the big steps forward has been the production of a new adhesive which bonds to the tooth and to the filling material, thus ensuring good retention and a watertight filling.

There is more use today of the special high-intensity lamps to 'set' these fillings and this gives the dentist more 'control', e.g. seeing that the material is correctly placed before applying a 'snap' set. One of the disadvantages of the composite fillings for posterior teeth (and they must be specially formulated for this area) is that the filling paste must be inserted in small increments, each portion being light cured for 20-40 seconds. Thus the insertion of each filling is fairly time-consuming and as the material is itself quite expensive the dentist's fee will probably be high.

It is worth repeating that if your back teeth are filled quite satisfactorily with a metal filling you should 'leave well alone'. It is unlikely that any ethical dentist will try to persuade you to have all your 'good' metal fillings removed and replaced by 'white' fillings. If there is any doubt it is wise to seek a second opinion.

The advent of these adhesive varnishes and fillings has had one beneficial effect. This is the new teaching of cavity preparation in which much smaller cavities are advocated, i.e. with considerably less 'drilling'.

Dentists are now becoming much more concerned with cosmetic dentistry because they have so many possibilities of matching almost any shade with composites and porcelains. Some good cosmetic results can be obtained with the minimum of drilling.

Local anaesthetics (injections)

A new type of local anaesthesia syringe is being used by some dentists, in a new technique called intraligamentary injection. In this a very fine needle is used attached to the special syringe which emits only a few drops of anaesthetic at a time. The needle is passed between the gum and the tooth and does not pierce the gums from the surface. It is quite comfortable and many dentists have had favourable results with this method. The dentists who do not use this technique find that their own standard technique gives the same results; however it is almost impossible for any dentist to give a 'clumsy' injection with the intraligamentary syringe. The bigger advantage, though, is the fact that only very small amounts of anaesthetic are used; thus the recovery of the mouth after treatment is quicker and there rarely is that 'dead' feeling to the lips and tongue as with the conventional syringe.

X-rays

The speed of X-ray films has been increased considerably (matching the fast films now common in photography). This means that the X-ray machine is 'on' for a shorter time and some exposures are in the region of ¼ second or less. The *much wider use* of panoramic X-ray examinations has also meant lower X-ray dosage combined with ability to see structures which were not previously visible using conventional machines (see page 72).

Gum and periodontal disease

There is a tendency for less radical surgery to be carried out in many cases. That is, much less extensive cutting of the gums is being done.

The emphasis is on thorough cleansing, and the greater use of dental hygienists has had a great effect on preventing disease and its progression.

In very severe cases of periodontal disease it was estimated (page 33) that very small amounts of grafts may be used to fill in bone which had been lost from around the tooth. In fact it has always been a problem as to where this bone for grafting could be obtained and often it was taken from another part of the jaw. However, new synthetic materials are being used to fill the bone defects under the gum. The material is hydroxylapatite which looks like white sand. The composition of the material is very similar to that of dental enamel and has been very well tolerated in the mouth. The material has been used extensively in the USA and by some specialists in the UK. There is no doubt that it will soon be available in special practices.

Dentists and dental hygienists have been using ultrasonic methods for scaling the tartar from the teeth (page 30) and now it is possible that some will follow the scaling by finally polishing the teeth by using an air/water bicarbonate jet. This can very effectively remove difficult stains on teeth especially at hard-to-reach pits and fissures on the surface.

Because it is expensive, it is reasonable to expect that not all dentists will possess such equipment and therefore they will carry out the polishing with rubber cups or little brushes and paste. This is just as effective but may take longer.

Dentures

Complete dentures are being made with plastic materials which have far more resistance to fracture. We are therefore seeing fewer emergencies with broken dentures, but these will occur occasionally. It is always wise, if it is economically possible, to have a spare set made and it is especially important to take these on holidays or trips away from home.

Sometimes, because of shrinkage of the jaws upon which the denture should rest (usually the lower), it becomes impossible to retain it in place – and also there may be pain due to pressure on nerves. The artificial bone material (hydroxylapatite, previously mentioned) is being used to build up the bone height. This material is injected (as a mass of tiny beads under the surface of the gum covering the jaws) and moulded into shape. After about six weeks new dentures can be made. It is probable that this type of bone replacement will be available in the near future.

Dentifrices

These seem to be changing and improving regularly and so it makes recommendation of any particular brand difficult because replacement soon takes place. About 95 per cent of all toothpaste sold contains fluoride, and much of the improved dental health in children is associated with this increased use.

Fixed bridgework

In some cases, where there are just a few teeth missing (or a single tooth), it may be possible to make a fixed replacement without the necessity of extensive drilling of the teeth on either side to take crowns which support the bridge. The new bridgework goes by the name of Rochette or Maryland and the teeth are fixed to a metal frame which is specially treated to be attached to the supporting teeth with adhesive resin bond.

The advantage, of course, is preservation of the adjoining teeth with very little drilling, if any, and an obvious reduction in cost. A similar technique can be used for splinting loose teeth where this is necessary.

Some Common Dental Terms

Abscess	A collection of pus in a cavity. The result of infection, it can be *acute* (sudden and painful) or *chronic* (often not noticed by the patient).
Abutment tooth	A tooth used as a support to hold a bridge or false tooth.
Ache	A dull pain generally continuous.
Acrylic resin	A form of plastic (resin) from which some teeth and dentures are made.
Align (or aline)	To arrange the teeth in a normal line.
Alveolus	The jawbone around the root of the tooth. Hence *alveolar* relating to the alveolus.
Amalgam	A metal used for filling teeth. It is inserted in a plastic state and hardens rapidly. It is made from silver, tin and other metals such as copper, mixed before use with mercury.
Amputation	The surgical removal of part of the tooth usually referring either to the pulp (nerve) or the root.
Anaesthesia	Loss of feeling. Anaesthesia may be *local* (by injection) or *general* (of the whole body by inhalation or injection of some anaesthetic agent). *Surface* anaesthesia; loss of sensation of the surface by applying a liquid or paste, usually before injection.
Analgesia	Insensitivity to pain. Analgesic: a pain reliever, e.g. aspirin.

Anterior	In front.
Anterior teeth	Incisors and canines.
Antibiotic	Substances usually derived from certain micro-organisms used to combat infection by other micro-organisms.
Antrum	An air cavity in the bone of the face, e.g. maxillary antrum or sinus.
Apex	The tip of the tooth furthest from the crown. (Adjective: apical.)
Aphthous Ulcer	A small ulcer in the mouth.
Apicectomy	The removal, by surgery, of the infected apex of the root.
Appliance	A plate or other construction in the mouth inserted for a special purpose, e.g. by orthodontists to move teeth.
Arch	The dental arch is a U-shaped arrangement of the teeth in upper and lower jaws.
Attrition	Wearing away, especially of the tooth crowns during chewing.
Bacillus	A rod-shaped micro-organism.
Bacteraemia	Bacteria in the bloodstream, usually for a short time.
Bacteria	Micro-organisms.
Bacterial endocarditis (sub-acute)	Bacteria growing inside part of the heart, usually streptococcus.
Benign	Not malignant, or not endangering life.
Biscuspid	A premolar, i.e. with two cusps.
Bifurcation	Division into two roots, often used for the area where they meet.
Bilateral	On both sides.
Biopsy	A microscopic examination of a piece of tissue taken from part of the body for diagnosis.
Bitewing	A special small X-ray film which is used to show only the crowns of the teeth to check for dental decay.
Bridge	Used to restore a missing tooth or teeth and is attached to natural teeth on either side.

	May be fixed or removable.
Buccal	Relating to the cheek.
Bur	A revolving cutting tool which is fitted into a dental handpiece to prepare cavities in teeth and for other purposes.
Calcification	Calcium salts deposited into softer substances causing hardening.
Calculus	A deposit of hard calcium salts on the teeth. (May also be an abnormal stone in such places as saliva duct or gall bladder, etc.)
Caries, dental	Decay of tooth substance.
Cautery	Used to destroy tissue by heat or chemical substance.
Cavity	A hollow caused by decay, or by the preparation before filling.
Cementum	Bone-like substance on the surface of the root of the tooth.
Cervical	The area around the tooth where the root joins the crown.
Clasp	A band, hook or wire which fastens a partial denture or orthodontic appliance to a natural tooth.
Cleft palate	A congenital defect with a varying sized gap in the palate.
Congenital	Condition present at birth. Often associated with cleft lip.
Curettage	Scraping away abnormal substance from the walls of periodontal pockets or from bony cavities.
Cusp	Pointed elevation on the biting surface of a tooth crown.
Cyst	A bag-like cavity or sac containing fluid or other abnormal substance.
Deciduous	Naturally shed, applied to baby or milk teeth.
Degeneration	Gradual breakdown of tissue usually without specific cause.
Dental floss	Waxed or unwaxed tape or silk thread to clean between teeth.

Dental plaque	A film of varying thickness made up mostly of bacteria firmly attached to the tooth when hygiene has been deficient.
Dental pulp	The soft tissue with blood vessels and nerves occupying the centre of the tooth, i.e. 'the nerve'.
Diastema	A space between two (usually front) teeth.
Disclosing solution or tablet	A staining material used in the mouth to show up plaque on the teeth.
Distal	Away from the midline of the mouth.
Edentulous	Without teeth.
Endodontics	Treatment of the dental pulp or root canal.
Endodontist	A specialist in root canal treatment.
Epithelium	A thin layer of cells covering the body and lining the gut, etc.
Erosion	Loss of some of the surface of the tooth due to action which may be chemical but is sometimes of uncertain origin.
Eruption	The emergence of a new tooth through the gum.
Fissure	A groove in the biting surface of the tooth.
Fissure sealant	A plastic material which is used to adhere to and close up the grooves in enamel surfaces.
Flap	A surgically raised area of tissue for access to the structures underneath.
Full denture	A denture replacing all the teeth in one jaw.
Gingiva	Gum tissue around the tooth.
Gingivitis	Inflammation of the gums.
Glossitis	Inflammation of the tongue.
Gumboil	An abscess associated with a tooth and presenting on the gum.
Haemostasis	Arrest of bleeding.
Halitosis	Unpleasant smelling breath.

Habsburg jaw	Greatly protruding lower jaw common to members of the ruling Habsburgs.
Hare (cleft) lip	Congenital failure to unite one or both sides of the upper lip. Often associated with cleft palate.
Headcap	Orthodontic harness fitting over the patient's head with attachments to move the jaws into a favourable position.
Impacted tooth	A tooth which is wedged so that it is unable to erupt.
Incisal edge	The cutting edge of a front tooth.
Inlay	A filling which is cast in metal, usually gold, from a wax pattern of the tooth cavity and is cemented into place.
Interdental	Between the teeth.
Intramuscular	Within a muscle. (As with an intramuscular injection.)
Intravenous	Into a vein.
Labial	Relating to the lips.
Lateral	To the side.
Lesion	An injury, defect, wound, breakdown or disease in a tissue.
Lingual	Relating to the tongue.
Malignant	Threatening life, as in cancer.
Malocclusion	Abnormal relationship of the jaws and teeth.
Mandible	The lower jaw.
Maxilla	The main bone of the upper jaw.
Medial	Towards the midline.
Mesial	Towards the midline of the dental arch.
Mucous membrane	The covering membrane of the cavities of the body which communicate with the exterior.
Occlusion	The meeting of the upper and lower teeth.
Occlusal surface	The surface of the tooth which normally meets a similar surface in the opposing jaw.
Oedema	Swelling caused by abnormal collection of fluid in the tissues.
Oral	Relating to the mouth.

Orthodontics	Treatment of irregularities of the teeth and jaw relationship.
Paedodontics	The treatment of teeth and mouths of children.
Palate	Roof of the mouth.
Papilla, interdental	The triangle of gum immediately between two contacting teeth.
Periapical	Around the apex of the tooth.
Pericoronitis	Inflammation of the gum around a partly erupted tooth (usually a wisdom tooth).
Periodontal	Relating to the gums and supporting structures of the teeth.
Periodontal pack	The dressing covering the wound after gum surgery.
Periodontal pocket	The crevice between the margin of the gum and the tooth which has been abnormally deepened by disease.
Periodontitis	Periodontal disease, inflammation of the supporting structures of the teeth; an extension of gingivitis.
Plaque	See 'Dental plaque'.
Pontic	The false part of a bridge suspended from the natural abutment teeth.
Prosthesis	Appliance to replace missing teeth, e.g. a denture.
Prosthetics	Planning and construction of prostheses.
Pulp chamber	The cavity at the centre of the tooth which leads into the root canal.
Pulpitis	Inflammation of the pulp (nerve) of the tooth.
Pyorrhoea	Flow of pus, but the term is used by members of the public to describe periodontal disease.
Quadrant	One quarter of the mouth, i.e. half of each dental arch, from the centre line to the last molar.
Radiography	The taking of images by X-rays and their interpretations.
Recession	The shrinking away of the gums revealing part of the root of the tooth.

Scaling	The removal of deposits, calculus, etc., from the teeth by the use of instruments.
Silicone	Elastic material used for impressions.
Silver point	Tapered fine cones used for filling root canals after the nerves have been removed.
Stump	That part of the tooth remaining after removal of the greater part of the crown.
Surface anaesthesia	Local anaesthesia produced by applying a solution to the surface before injection.
Suture	A stitch after surgery.
Temporomandibular joint	The articulating joint of the jawbone.
Thrush	An infection caused by a fungus – candida – characterized by white milky patches on the tongue and cheeks. Occurs more frequently in babies and old people and those who have been on prolonged antibiotic treatment.
Tartar	See 'Calculus'.
Trauma	An injury or wound.
'Trench Mouth'	Acute Ulcerative Gingivitis.
Tumour	An abnormal growth of tissue.
Ulcer	A localized break in the surface of the mouth (or skin), e.g. an open sore.
Unilateral	Occurring on one side only.
'Vincent's infection'	Acute Ulcerative Gingivitis (Necrotizing Ulcerative Gingivitis).
Wisdom tooth	Third molar.

Index